STOMACH DISORDERS

Edited by **Jianyuan Chai**

Stomach Disorders
http://dx.doi.org/10.5772/66029
Edited by Jianyuan Chai

Contributors

Wei Kang, Ka Fai To, Jinglin Zhang, Saheed Sabiu, Emmanuel Oladipo Ajani, Taofik Olatunde Sunmonu, Fatai Oladunni Balogun, Anofi Omotayo Tom Ashafa, Samia Gamie, Marcia Helena Braga Catroxo, Ana Maria Cristina Rebello Pinto Da Fonseca Martins, Daryl Ramai, Madhavi Reddy, Sandar Linn, Jianyuan Chai

Published by InTech
Janeza Trdine 9, 51000 Rijeka, Croatia

Publishing Process Manager Maja Bozicevic
Technical Editor SPi Global
Cover InTech Design team

First published January, 2018
Printed in Croatia
Legal deposit, Croatia: National and University Library in Zagreb

Additional hard copies can be obtained from orders@intechopen.com

Stomach Disorders, Edited by Jianyuan Chai
p. cm.
Print ISBN 978-953-51-3728-3
Online ISBN 978-953-51-3729-0

For EU product safety concerns:
IN TECH d.o.o., Prolaz Marije Krucifikse Kozulić 3, 51000 Rijeka, Croatia,
info@intechopen.com or visit our website at intechopen.com.

Meet the editor

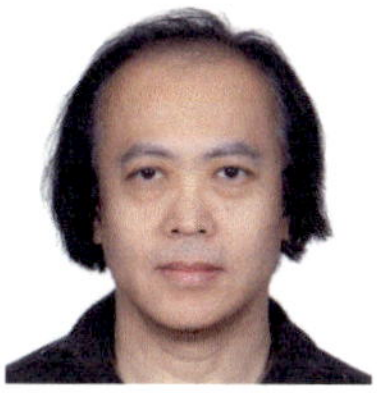

Dr. Chai received his PhD degree from the City University of New York in 1998 and completed his postdoctoral training at Harvard University in 2001. Then he served the Department of Veterans Affairs of the United States as a Principal Investigator (2002–2016), in affiliation with the School of Medicine, University of California, in Irvine. Currently, he is a professor at Baotou Medical College, Inner Mongolia University of Science and Technology. He has published dozens of research articles on various subjects including zoology, cardiovascular biology, gastroenterology, and cancer biology. In addition, he holds membership with AGA, AHA, ASBMB and other professional organizations, has served on the editorial board of multiple journals, and has also been a solicited reviewer for national and international funding agencies.

Contents

Preface

The stomach is one of the most critical organ in our body and is also the one that suffers most, because it carries many burdens in addition to its own duty. Our biological body relies on two sources of supply from the environment: oxygen taken in through the respiratory system and food through the digestive tract. While breathing is an involuntary action, meaning that the body does it automatically without our effort, eating is not. If we do not eat actively, we will die of starvation. The Chinese has an old saying, "Living is for eating and wearing," and another one goes like this, "Eating and sleeping are essential for life." They both recognize the importance of eating. In modern civilization, eating is no longer just a way to provide nutritional supply to the body. It has become an entertainment activity as well. We like to entertain our taste buds with various food, all sorts of flavors, and sometimes even try some exotics just for fun. We eat French cuisine today and perhaps Italian tomorrow; Kentucky fried chicken for lunch, and perhaps Korean barbecue for dinner. As a result, our stomach has to learn to deal with all of these frequent changes. One might say, "That's a duty for being a digestive organ. What else do you expect?" Well, let's say this is true. We must eat when we are hungry, but what about drinking? Every time when we are thirsty, we will let the stomach carry a load of liquid. If it is just water, that would be fine too. But, a lot of people are carelessly pouring whisky or vodka down the throat. These beverages contain at least 40% ethanol and can damage the stomach lining and cause gastritis, ulceration, or even gastric malignancy. What is even worse is smoking. Supposedly smoking ought to be a job for the respiratory system, but part of our digestive system (mouth and esophagus at least) has to suffer from it as well. Smoking can not only weaken the lower esophageal sphincter and allow acid reflux to happen but can also reduce mucus secretion in the stomach and elevate the risk of gastric ulcers or even cancer. That's not all. Every time when we are sick, we feed the stomach with all kinds of drugs regardless whether it is a stomach problem. Moreover, some people have no self-control over food. They keep eating and eating and eventually become obese, but they blame the stomach for it. They either have their stomachs tightened up with a band (gastric band) or have a slice cut off (sleeve gastrectomy). Even after all these, our stomach still keeps doing its job day and night dutifully and makes sure our body gets the best quality supplies that this organ can possibly provide.

The stomach is commonly known as a digestive organ; however, as pointed out in Chapter 1, its functions are far beyond simple digestion. First, the stomach is a place for food storage, and for this reason, we do not need to eat frequently in order to maintain health. This allows us to be able to concentrate on our work for hours without being distracted by food consumption. The stomach can also act as the first line of defense for our body by sterilizing the food that we have swallowed. Although the food has been passing through the mouth and the esophagus before reaching the stomach, these two parts of the digestive system do not have sophisticated defense mechanisms, and the food only stays in there briefly. The true interface between our internal biological machinery and the external world is our stomach. Once the food gets into the stomach, the stomach keeps the food inside for several hours and washes the food with its highly acidic juice up and down, back and forth, making sure there is no chance for any pathogens to go further into the rest of our body.

Among all the cancers known so far, gastric cancer is ranked globally as number five by its prevalence and number three by its mortality. Like other digestive disorders, gastric cancer is more common in developing countries, particularly in East Asia and Eastern Europe. Among all the risk factors, *Helicobacter pylori* infection has been found to be the predominant one. Considering the fact that more than half of the world population is carrying this bacterium, we can imagine the risk of stomach cancer. Over 90% of gastric malignancies are adenocarcinoma, which develops from the glandular epithelial cells. Chapter 2, "Molecular Pathogenesis of Gastric Adenocarcinoma," written by scholars from the Chinese University of Hong Kong, gives us an update about this disease from molecular perspective and raises several interesting questions about molecules involved in the cancer development and their therapeutic potential. It opens up some urgent areas for us to dig deeper.

There are many disorders associated with the stomach, but gastric ulcer is the most common chronic infection in the entire human population. Although it mainly affects the developing countries, it can be found in other regions of the world as well. *Helicobacter pylori* infection has been blamed for the majority of cases; therefore, eradication of the bacterium has helped to control the disease significantly. However, the stomach lumen contains some powerful harsh agents (such as hydrochloric acid and pepsin) that can cause ulceration whenever there is a chance for them to make a direct contact with the gastric epithelium. For this reason, any damages to the mucous layer of the stomach can be opportunities for ulcers to develop. The long-term use of nonsteroidal anti-inflammatory drugs (NSAIDs) creates such opportunities. NSAIDs function as pain relievers by inhibiting cyclooxygenase (COX), which is responsible for the synthesis of prostaglandin. Without adequate prostaglandin, the mucous layer cannot be renewed as it is needed periodically, and as a consequence, the gastric mucosa becomes vulnerable for any harsh agents. People have a long history of using various plants or their derivatives to treat stomach ulcers. Chapter 3, "The Purview of Phytotherapy in the Management of Gastric Ulcer," contributed by our African colleagues, broadens the topic further by reviewing nearly 70 species of plants that have been reported for their antiulcer effects. This is an excellent reference for people who are interested in some further studies on these plants, such as molecular mechanisms of their actions in gastric protection, etc.

Portal hypertensive gastropathy (PHG) and gastric antral vascular ectasia (GAVE) are two poorly studied conditions, basically referring to two types of gastritis in patients with portal hypertension. However, their pathophysiology and treatment options are different. It should be clear that not all portal hypertension patients will develop PHG or GAVE definitely. PHG only happens to 20–75% of portal hypertension patients. They both can cause gastric bleeding and other complications. As portal hypertension is mainly caused by cirrhosis, both PHG and GAVE are frequently found in association with liver cirrhosis. In Chapters 4 and 5, Dr. Ramai, Linn, and Reddy (Brooklyn Hospital Center, USA, and St George's University School of Medicine, Grenada) and Dr. Gamie (Helwan University, Egypt) update us with a detailed review on these rare diseases. Reading through these papers gives you an urgent feeling for more study, because the available data are just too inconclusive.

Gastroenteritis, commonly known as the "stomach flu," is an infectious disease, although it has nothing to do with influenza. It is mainly caused by viruses, especially rotavirus, which is responsible for about 70% of the patients, but other pathogens like bacteria, parasites, and even fungi can induce gastroenteritis as well. Children are the main targets, especially in developing countries. In the United States, gastroenteritis represents the second most common infection after the common cold. Among 2 billion cases worldwide in the year 2015, 1.3 million were dead, and most of them were children under five. Although we were unable to include an essay on human gastroenteritis in this book, Chapter 6, "Application of Transmission Electron Microscopy Techniques in the Veterinary Diagnosis of Viral Gastroenteritis in Livestock Animals," contributed by Catroxo and Martins, introduces the disease in livestock and gives a detailed description on how to use electron microscope to identify the pathogens. Coincidently, rotavirus was also found as the main cause of animal gastroenteritis. Therefore, this work remains valuable to our human studies. Besides, electron microscopic technique is universal. In order to make the best vaccines for this disease, identification of the pathogens is critical. Transmission electron microscopy has been proved to be a reliable method to do the job.

We can choose what to eat, when to eat, and how to eat. However, whatever we eat, the stomach is the first station to store it, to inspect it, to process it, and finally to issue a pass for its next journey. Without a healthy stomach, we cannot have a happy life. So, please take good care of it.

Jianyuan Chai, PhD
Baotou Medical College, China
University of California, USA

Chapter 1

Introductory Chapter: Stomach-Beyond Digestion

Jianyuan Chai

Additional information is available at the end of the chapter

http://dx.doi.org/10.5772/intechopen.72520

1. Introduction

The human body essentially relies on two sources to provide energy and building blocks, oxygen and food. The oxygen is taken in through the respiratory system and can be utilized almost directly for metabolic reactions, while food, after eaten, has to be sent on to a long journey of digestion before becoming utilizable nutrients to nurture the body. This heavy lifting is done by the digestive system. According to the World Health Organization (WHO), more than 6 million people on earth die of various digestive disorders every year [1], only second to heart disease (~7 million). Therefore, it is absolutely vital to understand how this system works and to take good care of it.

The human digestive system is more or less a 9-m long tube starting from the mouth and ending at the anus, plus some accessary glands including liver, pancreas, and gallbladder. The food is first chewed in the mouth, then swallowed down through the esophagus, and stays in the stomach for several hours, depending on the nature of the food and the motility of the organ, before it is sent to the small intestine to be extracted. The word *stomach* is originally derived from the Greek word *stomachos*, *stoma* meaning "mouth." It is essentially an enlargement of the digestive tract between the esophagus and the duodenum. We also frequently use the word *gastric* when we talk about stomach-related issues, and the word *gastric* is derived from the Greek word *gaster*, meaning "belly."

The stomach is separated from the rest of the body by two muscular rings, which keep the stomach contents contained. The lower esophageal sphincter, at the junction of the esophagus and the stomach, prevents the highly acidic gastric materials from backing up into the esophagus, otherwise esophageal damages may occur; while the pyloric sphincter, at the junction of the stomach with the duodenum, controls the amount of partially digested food to go into the duodenum, giving the small intestines enough time to absorb as much nutrients from the food as possible. The stomach sends food into the duodenum only when the intestine is not occupied.

The stomach is commonly known as a digestive organ. Although the major digestive events take place in the small intestines where multiple enzymes meet their right conditions, the process of digestion actually begins at the moment of eating. Chewing is a form of mechanical digestion, which crushes the food from big pieces into smaller ones, and the saliva contains digestive enzymes like amylase and lipase, which can break down carbohydrates and lipids. The stomach represents the second phase of digestion, which breaks down proteins into small peptides and thereby facilitates the intestinal digestion. Like the other parts of the digestive tract, the human stomach wall is structurally made of mucosa, submucosa, muscularis externa, and serosa at the histological level. The gastric mucosa consists of the simple columnar epithelium, some loose connective tissue called the lamina propria, and a thin layer of smooth muscle called the muscularis mucosae, which separate the mucosa from the submucosa beneath. At the cellular level, there are several types of secreting cells embedded within the gastric epithelium. The outermost surface of the stomach is lined with the foveolar cells, which produce alkaline mucus for shielding the epithelium from the stomach acid. The stomach has to regenerate a new layer of mucus every 2 weeks, otherwise damage to the epithelium may occur. The parietal cells, mainly found in the fundus and the stomach body, are responsible for making hydrochloric acid to sterilize the food that is brought in by the esophagus. In addition, the parietal cells also make a glycoprotein called intrinsic factor, which is required for vitamin B12 absorption. Then, the chief cells, located in the deep mucosa, produce an enzyme precursor called pepsinogen. Only in the acidic environment, this molecule can become the active enzyme pepsin for proteolysis. The production of hydrochloric acid is regulated by a hormone called gastrin, which is secreted by another type of cells called G cells. The G cells are usually located in the middle portion of the pyloric glands and are occasionally also seen in the duodenum and pancreas. All of these endocrinal cells coordinately work together for digestion. Basically, once the stomach is filled with food, the G cells start to secrete gastrin to stimulate the release of hydrochloric acid from the parietal cells and pepsinogen from the chief cells. Hydrochloric acid then converts pepsinogen into pepsin, which ultimately breaks down proteins into small peptides readily for the small intestines to absorb or to process further.

Pepsin is one of three proteases that we have for protein digestion, and the other two, trypsin and chymotrypsin, are both derived from the pancreas. When the mucous coating of the stomach is damaged by bacterial infection or drugs use, pepsin can reach the gastric epithelium and cause gastritis or ulceration. Overproduction of hydrochloric acid can also cause gastric ulcers. Zollinger-Ellison syndrome is a good example, in which ulcerations develop in the stomach due to tumor-related excessive gastrin release. Gastrin increases both the number of parietal cells and the production of hydrochloric acid [2]. As a result, the mucous layer could not deal with the overwhelming acidity and eventually gives in, then ulceration takes place.

For people who have gastroesophageal reflux disease (GERD), pepsin can be brought up into the esophagus along with the stomach acid to cause esophagitis or esophageal ulcers. If it goes up further into the larynx or pharynx, laryngitis or pharyngitis may occur. Chronic reflux is also possible to induce bronchitis or pneumonia. GERD is the most common gastrointestinal diagnosis given during office visits. In the United States, the overall costs of GERD management exceed $85 billion a year [3, 4]. Today, over 60% of Americans experience occasional episodes of acid reflux, and about 25% have to deal with the problem on a weekly basis [5]. Current GERD treatment primarily relies on acid-suppressive medications. However, inhibition of acid secretion can cause various digestive disorders, because hydrochloric acid is an essential element for the stomach to function normally. People who have received this type of treatment have shown multiple side effects such as diarrhea, constipation, decreased absorption of vitamins/minerals, and susceptibility to bacterial infections, bone fracture, and even elevated risk of cancer [6]. Over the years, the Food and Drug Administration of the United States has issued warnings repeatedly against this type of drugs.

In addition to digestion, the stomach can also function as a place for absorption. Although the main absorption in the human digestive system takes place in the small intestine, some small molecules nevertheless can be picked up in the stomach through its lining. This includes water, medication, amino acids, alcohol, caffeine, and some water-soluble vitamins.

The second important function of the stomach is for storage. In the animal kingdom, there is not always plenty of food available to eat or to obtain easily. Very often animals have to risk their lives to fight for a meal. Death due to starvation is very common in the wild world. During the history of evolution, animals learned to adapt this situation by developing an internal pouch to store extra food that they had acquired, so that they could stay alive for a period of time without constant hunting and eating. This structure is the stomach. In some animals, like ruminants, this organ can be very fancy and complicated. For this type of animals, every meal could be an adventure, a life-threatening event, because they usually do not possess excellent fighting skills to protect themselves against predators. Consequently, they have developed a big stomach that is able to hold a large quantity of food. For example, the stomach of a cow can retain 95 l of undigested materials. When they are in a safe place, they can regurgitate the food from the stomach and chew it more slowly and efficiently. The human stomach, on the other hand, is relatively small and can only hold up to 1 l of food. Because human beings have been more skillful survivors by nature comparing to other animals, and they do not always have to face the danger in order to feed themselves, carrying a big stomach would be a burden to them. Nevertheless, the human stomach has experienced the same path of evolution anyhow. Although they do not need to store a lot of food internally for survival, having a food pocket like the stomach has still made their lives much easier. In a modern civilized society, most people eat only 2–4 meals a day, and sometimes eating to them is not for hungry but just a social activity for pleasure. This allows them to be able to spend the rest of the day doing other things, such as listening to music, playing tennis, or walking on the beach. Even if you have to rush to work after eating, having such an internal pocket to save a big steak or a milkshake is amazing.

However, when the stomach has storage issues, the life of the patient can be problematic. For instance, for people with gastric cancer or severe gastric perforation, their stomach has to be removed partially or completely through gastrectomy, consequently, they will have to eat more frequently in order to uptake adequate nutrition. On the other hand, for people with obesity, to help them to lose weight, a gastric band may be placed around the cardia area to reduce the stomach capacity or to bypass the stomach entirely, so that they will not be able to eat as much as they used to. However, after this kind of surgeries, a condition called dumping syndrome may develop, in which patients experience abdominal cramps or diarrhea soon after eating, especially for food containing high level of carbohydrates, because the small bowel is not made to handle the food rush without a proper preparation and regulation by the stomach [7].

Defense is another important function of the stomach that should not be overlooked. As we said at the beginning, there are two major passageways through which the human body actively takes in raw materials from the environment, oxygen through the respiratory system and food through the digestive system. As a result, these two passageways become the easiest routes for pathogens to invade our body. The Chinese has an old saying, "Illnesses are all derived from the mouth." It tells some truth about the importance of our eating habits. During the history of evolution, the mankind has learned to cook, which has two purposes: one is to make the food easier to digest and absorb after denaturation, and the second is to kill the pathogens hidden in the food. In the modern civilized world, most people primarily live on cooked food, but sometimes we like to taste the freshness of raw materials like fresh vegetables, fruits, and even raw meat occasionally. Although these goods have already been cleaned up before sold in the market, there are still a lot of people who have no access to these modern hygienic facilities. They eat whatever harvested directly from the field or leftovers without the necessary heating-up. These life styles have accidentally turned on the green light to the pathogens. One-third of the world's digestive fatalities is caused by diarrhea, making it the most common digestive disorder in the undeveloped regions. For instance, in Angola, diarrhea is responsible for more than 17% of the total number of annual deaths. Fortunately, our digestive system has evolved with some fantastic defense mechanisms. If the food does not taste right, we can get it out of our system by spitting or vomiting. However, our taste buds cannot always distinguish whether there are pathogens in the food. For most of the time after eaten, it is up to the stomach to deal with whatever comes next. Thankfully, we have an amazing stomach, which can function as a sterilizer by creating a highly acidic environment inside our body and keeping its acidity around pH 2.0 for most of the time. Pathogens can rarely survive through such a harsh condition [8]. That eliminates numerous risks we might have to deal with otherwise. So, we should be very careful when it comes to acid-suppressive treatment.

Author details

Jianyuan Chai[1,2*]

*Address all correspondence to: jianyuan.chai@gmail.com

1 The Second Affiliated Hospital of Baotou Medical College, Inner Mongolia University of Science and Technology, Baotou, China

2 School of Medicine, University of California, Irvine, California, USA

References

[1] Chai J. Gastric ulcer healing—Role of serum response factor. In: Chai J, editor. Peptic Ulcer Disease. Rijeka: Intech Publisher; 2011. pp. 143-164. DOI: 10.5772/17410 ISBN: 978-953-307-976-9

[2] Smith JP, Nadella S, Osborne N. Gastrin and gastric cancer. Cellular and Molecular Gastroenterology and Hepatology. 2017;**4**:75-83. DOI: 10.1016/j.jcmgh.2017.03.004

[3] Shaheen NJ, Hansen RA, Morgan DR, Gangarosa LM, Ringel Y, Thiny MT, Russo MW, Sandler RS. The burden of gastrointestinal and liver diseases. The American Journal of Gastroenterology. 2006;**101**:2128-2138. DOI: 10.1111/j.1572-0241.2006.00723.x

[4] Walqvist P, Reilly MC, Barkun A. Systematic review: The impact of gastro-oesophageal reflux disease on work productivity. Alimentary Pharmacology & Therapeutics. 2006;**24**:259-272. DOI: 10.1111/j.1365-2036.2006.02996.x

[5] Chai J, Jamal MM. Esophageal malignancy—A growing concern. World Journal of Gastroenterology. 2012;**18**:6521-6526. DOI: 10.3748/wjg.v18.i45.6521

[6] Chubineh S, Birk J. Proton pump inhibitors: The good, bad, and the unwanted. Southern Medical Journal. 2012;**105**:613-618. DOI: 10.1097/SMJ.0b013e31826efbea

[7] Camilleri M, Malhi H, Acosta A. Gastrointestinal complications of obesity. Gastroenterology. 2017;**152**:1656-1670. DOI: 10.1053/j.gastro.2016.12.052

[8] Hunt RH, Camilleri M, Crowe SE, El-Omar EM, Fox JG, Kuipers EJ, Malfertheiner P, McColl KE, Pritchard DM, Rugge M, Sonnenberg A, Sugano K, Tack J. The stomach in health and disease. Gut. 2015;**64**:1650-1668. DOI: 10.1136/gutjnl-2014-307595

Chapter 2

Molecular Pathogenesis of Gastric Adenocarcinoma

Wei Kang, Jinglin Zhang and Ka Fai To

Additional information is available at the end of the chapter

http://dx.doi.org/10.5772/intechopen.69951

Abstract

The incidence and mortality of gastric cancer (GC) rank top five and top three, respectively, among cancers around the world. It is an intricate malignancy caused by the reciprocity of intrinsically genetic, environmental, and host-related elements. The silent property, advanced clinical characterization, and potential heterogeneity have made GC a thorny disease with a high death rate. The increasing knowledge of the abundant genetic abnormalities regarding GC will definitely elongate the patients' survival. Scientists have been working hard to discover the myths beneath gastric tumorigenesis: novel biomarkers have been established, and cell transduction cascades have been well described. The study grouping GC into four molecular subtypes by The Cancer Genome Atlas (TCGA) broadens our horizon of GC etiologies. Knowledge regarding to the sophisticated networks in tumor microenvironment also bring new insights into the mechanisms assist GC development. In the future, people will strive for translating more research achievements into clinical utility. Successful translational medicine will lead to new methods for early GC diagnosis and precise medical strategies for individuals.

Keywords: gastric adenocarcinoma, molecular classification, pathogenesis

1. Introduction

Gastric cancer (GC) is the fifth most common malignancy worldwide and third leading cancer-related death. Because of poor diagnosis, 5-year survival rate of GC is rather low, ranging from 15 to 52% [1, 2]. The incident rates are higher in men than in women. GC contributes over 20% of morbidity and mortality to cancer all over the world annually, following lung and liver cancer, which account for 23 and 28%, respectively. In 2012, approximate 723,000 deaths and more than 950,000 new GC cases were reported worldwide. Despite the incidence of GC has been declining in the North American and most of the west European countries, GC remains a type of prevailing cancer with increasing risk in regions including

Asia, Eastern Europe, and certain areas of Latin America [3]. Particularly, adenocarcinomas, which developed from the glands of the most superficial layer or the mucosa, take up 90% of GC. The rest types of GC include mucosa-associated lymphoid tissue (MALT) lymphomas, which originate from the muscles surrounding mucosa areas of the stomach [4].

The risk factors include environmental factors, such as *Helicobacter pylori* infection, cigarettes smoking and high-salt diet, and host genetic alterations. Although the incidence of GC has shown a dramatic decrease in recent years due to *H. pylori* eradication, the overall survival is still quite poor due to its silent nature, late clinical presentation, and genetic heterogeneity. Thus, comprehensive understanding of the detailed molecular mechanisms and accurate pathogenesis of GC will improve patient outcome. Recently, several kinds of molecular classification of GC have been provided to reveal the genomic landscape of GC and decipher the crucial molecular changes. Among them, The Cancer Genome Atlas (TCGA) classification is a milestone for the molecular characterization of GC. Clinical translation of these molecular findings will provide novel strategies for early GC detection and promote precision therapies for GC patients.

2. The risk factors of GC

GC is defined as a tumor with multifactorial etiologies. Environmental alteration and genetic factors play major roles in GC, particularly, virus infection, dietary habits, and lifestyles are recognized to be critical factors.

H. pylori is a common human pathogen, contributing to both malignant and benign diseases. Among all the risk factors of GC, *H. pylori* is considered to be the most predominant factor, up to 80% of GC cases are led by *H. pylori* infection. At least 660,000 new diagnoses are making annually [5, 6]. Data in western countries indicated that *H. pylori* is a major risk factor for only non-cardia GC instead of cardia GC [5]. It has been noted that the death number of GC is decreasing in many developed regions, partially related to eradication therapy and improved living condition in certain populations and regions [7]. Given the worldwide aging problem and the migration trend of people from high to low prevalence regions, the mortality is very likely to increase in the future [8]. *H. pylori* infection alone is not sufficient to trigger GC. Chiba et al. suggested *H. pylori* infection contributed to GC development via two potential mechanisms, either caused chronic inflammation or directly acted on epithelial cells [9]. In general, *H. pylori* colonizes the gastric mucosal epithelium and induces chronic inflammation at the beginning of infection, while persistent inflammation resulted in GC [10, 11]. Cytokines and chemokines produced by the tumor microenvironment facilitate cell proliferation and migration, and keep cells from apoptosis and immune detection [12]. Cytokines released by different cell sources have been described as suggestive indicators in the progression of GC. The serum level of Tumor necrosis factor-α (TNF--α) in GC was found greatly reduced, however, levels of TNF-α in stage III or IV GC patients showed a significant elevation when compared to levels in earlier stage patients [13]. Besides, the secretion of Interleukin-1 (IL-1) contributes to tumor cell proliferation and progression. In addition, IL-6, IL-10, and Transforming growth factor-β (TGF-β) improve survival of GC cells by promoting cell invasion and suppression of antitumor immunity. IL-11, IL-17, IL-18, IL-22, and chemokines secreted by a specific cell type also improve the progression of GC [14]. Major types of virulence factors of *H. pylori* include cytotoxin VacA, the type IV secretion system (T4SS), and the CagA effector protein. These factors are associated with multiple cellular responses, such as induction of oxidative stress and epithelial barrier disruption, in various model systems [15].

Epstein-Barr virus (EBV), also termed as human herpesvirus 4 (HHV-4), is one of the most prevalent viruses in humans. EBV was the first virus identified in human carcinoma in 1964 [16]. Approximately 95% of adults in the world are infected by EBV due to the positive detection of serological EBV markers. EBV infection may not cause severe symptoms and disease. After primary infection, EBV establishes a carrier state called latent stage. However, latent EBV infection could subsequently become high-risk oncogenic factors associated with human malignancies. EBV has been known as another significant pathogen exists in GC cells. According to worldwide data, EBV-associated GC (EBVaGC) accounts for 10%, in average, of total GC cases. Most of the EBVaGC cases were epithelial tumors, while lymphoepithelioma-like carcinomas take up 90% of the rest rare EBVaGC cases. EBVaGC presents distinct clinic properties, such as predominance among male and younger individuals and predominant proximal stomach location [17]. EBV infection can be achieved by two different entry mechanisms, either via B cell entry or fusion with epithelial cells directly [18, 19]. EBVaGC occurs in the upper and middle stomach in the majority. Fukayama et al. indicated the tumor distribution in the stomach, with the proportion that 58% in the cardia, 33% in the body, and 9% in the antrum [20, 21]. They also depicted the appearance of EBVaGC as ulcerated or saucer-like, with obvious thickened gastric wall. Moreover, the lymph node was less frequently involved during early stage within the submucosa. These characteristics are proposed to be favorable prognosis indicators. Histological studies provide evidence that immune cell infiltration was a feature of EBVaGC. For instance, infiltrating lymphocytes, containing EBV-specific cytotoxic T cells, communicate with carcinoma cells directly, in the opposite, cytokine IL-1β was upregulated to recruit noninfiltrating lymphocytes against this cell-cell contact [22, 23]. Therefore, in EBVaGC, immune responses in tumor microenvironment also accompany with the progression of EBVaGC [24].

Dietary factors: dietary risks, including salty and spicy food intake, cigarettes smoking, frequent coffee, and high-temperature drinking habits are positively associated with GC. Intriguingly, excess salt intake showed susceptibility to EBVaGC and *H. pylori*-induced GC. Habitual excess salt intake was suggested to progressively increase the risk across consumption levels of GC via a meta-analysis [25]. The association between salty food intake and *H. pylori* infection was also evaluated in a cross-sectional study of 634-middle age male cohort. The result supported habitual salt-rich Japanese food intake was prevalent in *H. pylori*-induced GC cases [26]. It is probably due to the increase of *H. pylori* colonization and persistent infection [27]. Besides salty food intake, Camargo et al. indicated that smoking was strongly associated with EBVaGC by a case-case comparison between EBV-positive tumors and EBV-negative tumors [28]. Although alcohol drinking was a suggestive risk factor of GC, heavy alcohol drinking, rather than moderate alcoholic drinks, was significantly correlated with GC development [29, 30].

3. Molecular classification and pathogenies of GC

Up to 90% of stomach malignancies are adenocarcinomas. Non-Hodgkin's lymphomas and gastrointestinal stromal tumor (GIST) make up most of the remaining 10% [31]. Even though infrequently, adenosquamous, squamous, and undifferentiated carcinomas also occur. In regard to clinical diagnosis, several pathological characterization varied from time to time. Several histological classification systems for gastric adenocarcinoma have been described, but the most frequently used are those of the World Health Organization (WHO) and Lauren [32]. In the World Health Organization (WHO) classification, there are 10 histological types [33]. The Lauren classification is commonly applied and it makes the distinction between intestinal and diffuse types. The intestinal GC consists of cohesive neoplastic cells forming gland-like structures while the diffuse type has lost cell cohesion and resulting in diffuse discohesive cellular infiltration [31]. Men and elderly are more likely to suffer intestinal type, whereas diffuse type carcinomas are relatively more common among the younger population with an equal male-to-female ratio [32]. Recently, a project named The Cancer Genome Atlas (TCGA) has proposed a brand new classification, in which GC is grouped by four subtypes: EBV-positive (EBV), microsatellite instability (MSI), genomically stable [34], and chromosomal instability [35, 36].

According to previous studies, about 9% of GC cases are infected by EBV [37]. All the EBV-positive GCs harbor the property of CpG island methylator phenotype (CIMP) [36, 38, 39]. EBV-positive tumors exhibited a higher incidence of whole-genomic DNA hypermethylation than any molecular subtypes. The genes with promoter hypermethylation showed most differentially silenced expression in EBV-associated GC [36]. Moreover, PI(3)-kinase inhibition was also strongly detected in EBV-positive GC, which offered a new method for the evaluation of this subtype [36]. The most highly transcribed EBV viral, message RNAs (mRNAs) and microRNAs (miRNAs), fell within the BamH1A region of the viral genome and showed similar expression patterns across tumors [36]. The mutation rate of PIK3CA is exclusively high in EBV-positive gastric cancer compared with other molecular subtypes. The mutation rate of PIK3CA in this subtype is about 80 and 68% of the mutations belongs to recurrent mutation in this dataset. In contrast, in other molecular subtypes, the mutation rates of PIK3CA are from 3 to 42%. So, this result provides a hint that using PI3K inhibitor might have the clinical therapeutic potential for this kind of molecular subtype.

The next subtypes of GC are abundant in MSI, which display increased mutation rates (in major histocompatibility complex class I genes, including B2M and HLA-B) and hypermethylation (containing hypermethylation at the *MLH1* promoter). The most obvious difference between EBV-CIMP (CpG island methylator phenotype) and MSI-associated gastric-CIMP methylation profiles is that all EBV-positive gastric tumors show promoter hypermethylation of *CDKN2A* ($p16^{INK4A}$), but the *MLH1* hypermethylation was only detected in MSI-associated CIMP [38].

In genomically stable subtype, *RHOA* mutation was detected [36]. When binding with Guanosine-5'-triphosphate (GTP), RHOA behaves through a great number of downstream effectors, such as ROCK1, mDIA, and protein kinase N. This will lead to actin-myosin-dependent cell contractility and cellular motility [40, 41] and activation of STAT3 to promote carcinogenesis [42, 43]. Except from activating mDia or ROCK1, the *RHOA* mutation Y42C has been confirmed to attenuate the activationof protein kinase N. Because RHOA is strongly associated with cell motility, the *RHOA* mutations might contribute to the invasive growth patterns. In diffuse type GC or genomically stable GC, the lack of cellular cohesion is a hallmark for this diffuse phenotype. Apart from RHOA mutation, an inter-chromosomal translocation called CLDN18-ARHGAP26 fusion gene was identified. ARHGAP26 is a GTPase-activating protein that converts GTP-RHO to GDP-RHO and it is been reported to facilitate cellular motility. CLDN18 is a tight junction component that involves in cell adhesion. This fusion gene thus was thought to correlate with cell metastasis in this kind of molecular subtype.

With the somatic copy-number aberrations (SCNAs), the last group of GC was clustered as CIN subtype. In this subtype, a bunch of genes shows dysregulated, such as *TP53* mutations (in 71% of tumors) as well as *CDH1* somatic mutations (enriched in the genomically stable subtype, about 37% of cases).

4. The dysregulated miRNAs involved in GC

MicroRNAs (miRNAs) are one predominant category of small (roughly 20–30 nucleotides) non-coding RNAs that participate in gene expression and control [44]. Their effects are mostly lead to the degradation of message RNAs (mRNAs) or inhibitory of the translations, and subsequently affect a series of biological behaviors of cells, such as inflammation, cell proliferation, apoptosis and differentiation. In the nucleus, together with its cofactor Pasha (DGCR8), the RNase III enzyme Drosha cut out primary miRNA transcripts into a fragment of approximately 60 nucleotides named precursor miRNAs (pre-miRNAs), and initiate the biogenesis of miRNAs [45]. A cytoplasmic RNase III called Dicer will be responsible for the further processing of the pre-miRNAs and makes them mature after they are transported to the cytoplasm [46, 47]. A mature miRNA, with the length of about 18–24 nucleotides, is single-stranded, which can sometimes aim at multiple targets. These mature miRNAs always bind to the complementary sequences of targeted mRNAs directly to make mRNAs degrade or bind directly to 3′-untranslated regions (3′-UTR) of mRNAs to decrease their translation, so that miRNAs can exert their effects on regulating certain gene expression [44, 48]. Accordingly, miRNAs regulate at least 30% of genes of human as it is estimated [49].

In other words, miRNAs are capable of acting as a switch to control genes related to cell proliferation and apoptosis under pathogenic circumstances, consequently, they may have a chance to be involved in both cancer initiation and progression. It seems that no matter how clear the mechanism of malignancy behaviors or an effective therapy that might prevent tumorigenesis from the beginning, an increasing knowledge of these miRNAs is crucial. During the physiological periods, miRNAs present or absent in proper time of different stage of lives. However, they are produced abnormally in tumors, that the levels of some miRNAs are highly detected while some are lower or even none. Hence, those which are upregulated called onco-miRs, whereas the downregulated ones called tumor-suppressive miRNAs. As the names suggested, genes controlled by onco-miRs are oncogenes whose products may promote tumor cells in many aspects, whereas the opposite site of genes is tumor suppressive, which plays a role of inhibitor among the initiation or development of tumors (e.g., miR-15a and miR-16-1, which target a member of Hippo pathway called YAP1, are downregulated in GC) [50]. Thus, identifying the target genes of these miRNAs is crucial and it may lead us to a better understanding of the miRNAs themselves.

For example, miR-21 was the first miRNA which was influenced by *H. pylori*. In tissues of both GC and *H. Pylori* infection, it was highly detected [51, 52]. Several data have reported that this miRNA can be used as a biomarker in GC diagnosis in the clinic [53–55]. And most recently, a research conducted in China suggested this miR-21 to be a GC biomarker in both diagnosis and prognosis, for the reason that, besides the high levels found in tumor tissues compared with the normal ones, miR-21 was revealed to be associated with poor survivals in clinical patients [56]. Behind the phenomena, the molecular mechanism is still unclear in GC. In other types of cancer, however, such as colorectal cancer, miR-21 decreased the tumor suppressor protein programmed cell death 4 (PDCD4) and exhibited an oncogenic function [57]. Additionally, in nonsmall cell lung carcinoma, miR-21 was found to deregulate PTEN, a tumor suppressor, to promote carcinogenesis [58].

5. The tumor microenvironment and gastric carcinogenesis

More and more evidence supported the idea that not only malignant GC cells, but also those nonmalignant cells involved in the tumor microenvironment play indispensable roles throughout GC pathogenesis. Generally, nonmalignant cells participate in various mechanisms related to GC development, such as stromal interactions, angiogenesis, and some immune responses.

Stromal components, including fibroblasts and extracellular matrix (ECM) adjacent to cancer cells, create a suitable environment for GC development. Stromal fibroblasts are known to play a central role in tumor microenvironment by interacting with cancer cells [59, 60]. However, other than ordinary fibroblasts, cancer-associated fibroblasts (CAFs) undergo a phenotypic change into myofibroblasts. Also, CAFs exhibit distinct gene expression patents that pertain to aberrant cell growth, focal adhesion, and ECM remodeling [61]. The remodeling ECM promotes the survival ability and distant colonization cancer cells by synthesizing components, such as type I and type III collagens, fibronectins, tenascin, and versican [62–64], as well as proteases like urokinase, plasminogen activator, fibroblast activation protein (FAP), and matrix metalloproteinases (MMPs) [65–67]. These characteristics are usually associated with poor prognostics. Moreover, tumor-related stromal fibroblasts secrete small molecules, such as IL-6 to stimulate cell growth, as well as factors associated with TGF-β signaling, triggering epithelial-mesenchymal transition (EMT) [68–70].

Angiogenesis is also a pivotal process contributes to tumor progression. Cell population in GC tumor microenvironment regulates the density and architecture of new blood vessels by stimulating the proliferation and differentiation of myofibroblasts and vascular endothelial cells [71, 72]. The growing number of new vessels was reported to facilitate GC metastasis [73, 74]. To promote angiogenesis, GC cells provide numerous angiogenic factors, including VEGF, FGF-2, CXCL1, and Ang-2, to microenvironment [75–78]. It has been noted that high level of VEGF-A contributed to endothelium-dependent angiogenesis. VEGF-A signaling increased both the new blood vessel number and permeability in GC [79]. VEGF-A strongly promotes the angiogenesis and aggressive phenotype of human intestinal-type GC [80]. Bevacizumab is a specific antibody against VEGF-A, and dominantly regulates normal and pathological angiogenesis. Clinical trials of bevacizumab in phase II advanced GC suggested a satisfied curative effect [81]. Unfortunately, in the randomized phase III Avastin in Gastric Cancer (AVAGAST) study, the combination of chemotherapy and bevacizumab did not show a better overall survival extension in the first-line treatment when compared to advanced GC patients, who only subjected chemotherapy [82]. Intriguingly, REGARD and RAINBOW trials using VEGFR2 targeting antibody ramucirumab have also shown a significant increase in the overall survival of patients with advanced GC [83]. It can be partially explained by the geographical differences of GC patients.

Immune reactivity in GC development is based on various types of immune cells in different stages [84]. First, in eliminating stage, macrophages and dendritic cells recruit to secrete chemokines and cytokines, such as IL-12 and IFN-γ, to phagocytize and remove apoptotic cancer cells [85]. Cancer cells survived from elimination subsequently under equilibrium stage and adapted to immune-suppression. The number of tumor-infiltrating lymphocytes (TILs) was noted as independent predictors to evaluate lymph node metastasis and GC patient survival in this stage. Interestingly, TILs exert either oncogenic or tumor-suppressive influence in GC cells, attributing to their unique functions. In a recent report, tumor-associated macrophages with high levels of CD163 expression exhibited aggressive characteristics and expression of cancer stem cell markers in recurrent GC cases. $CD163^+$ macrophages might, therefore, related to independent worse prognosis [86]. T-lymphocyte subsets are also significant cell types associated with both early onset of tumor and tumor progression. It has been reported that the high ratio of $CD8^+$ cytotoxic TILs/$FOXP3^+$ regulatory T cells (Treg) correlated with high overall survival rate and good prognosis, especially in MSI gastric cancer [87, 88]. Eventually, cancer cells escape from immune responses.

Immunogenicity could be blunted by releasing cytokines including TGF-β, TNF-α, and IL-10. Therefore, cancer cells can evade the detection by immune effectors in the tumor microenvironment [89]. PD-1 is one of the most important receptors expressed by T cells and monocytes. PD-1 negatively regulates the effectors by binding to its ligands PD-L1 and PD-L2. Blocking PD-1/PD-L1 has been suggested as a promising immune-therapeutic option [90, 91]. The relationship between PD-L1 level and prognosis remains under debate, however, a recent meta-analysis pooled all present data and suggested PD-L1 to be a valuable prognostic indicator of GC patients by dividing patients into different groups [92].

Collectively, tumor microenvironment composed of multiple subjects, such as tumor stromal fibroblasts, lymphocytes, and angiogenic factors. All these components cooperate together, configuring a context for GC development.

6. Conclusion

There is still a large realm of the unknown area about GC pathogenies even though the related research studies have been going deeper and our horizon has been broadened in the past few years. Epigenetically, we are seeking to unravel the mechanisms of gastric tumorigenesis affected by chromatin remodeling. Besides, there are miRNAs, lncRNAs, and some other classic molecules that are involved in GC development, which requires a more detailed investigation regarding these aspects. The most crucially and urgently, we are struggling to explore specific and precise therapies for patients who are suffering or likely to suffer from GC, especially genomically stable GC (a type of GC with a high mortality).

When it comes to the novel small entities, there are even more issues waiting to be addressed, such as how lncRNAs interact with chromatin alterations during gastric carcinogenesis. Moreover, in addition to *H. pylori* and EBV, scientists have identified a wild variety of bacteria in the stomach through DNA sequencing. These uncultivatable bacteria have formed a complicated community and there are few clues about how they interact with *H. pylori* and host immunity during GC initiation and progression. In the early detection field, molecular findings may facilitate new approaches for diagnosing GC early, by identifying high-risk potential sufferers via the molecular features of precancerous lesions. Finally, therapeutic strategies need to be designed precisely for each GC subtypes, according to their somatic driver change of genome or tumor-associated cell compartments, such as stromal cells and tumor-infiltrating immune cells.

Acknowledgements

This work is supported by the General Research Fund (RGC Reference No. CUHK14114414 and CUHK14110016) from the Research Grants Council of Hong Kong.

Author details

Wei Kang*, Jinglin Zhang and Ka Fai To

*Address all correspondence to: weikang@cuhk.edu.hk

Department of Anatomical and Cellular Pathology, State Key Laboratory of Oncology in South China, State Key Laboratory of Digestive Diseases, The Chinese University of Hong Kong, Hong Kong SAR, PR China

References

[1] Marchet A, Mocellin S, Ambrosi A, Morgagni P, Vittimberga G, Roviello F, Marrelli D, de Manzoni G, Minicozzi A, Coniglio A, Tiberio G, Pacelli F, Rosa F, Nitti D. Validation of the new AJCC TNM staging system for gastric cancer in a large cohort of patients (n = 2,155): Focus on the T category. European Journal of Surgical Oncology. 2011;**37**:779-785

[2] Nashimoto A, Akazawa K, Isobe Y, Miyashiro I, Katai H, Kodera Y, Tsujitani S, Seto Y, Furukawa H, Oda I, Ono H, Tanabe S, Kaminishi M. Gastric cancer treated in 2002 in Japan: 2009 annual report of the JGCA nationwide registry. Gastric Cancer. 2013;**16**:1-27

[3] International Agency for Research on Cancer. GLOBOCAN Database. IARC; 2008

[4] Karimi P, Islami F, Anandasabapathy S, Freedman ND, Kamangar F. Gastric cancer: Descriptive epidemiology, risk factors, screening, and prevention. Cancer Epidemiology Biomarkers & Prevention. 2014;**23**:700-713

[5] Helicobacter and Cancer Collaborative Group. Gastric cancer and Helicobacter pylori: a combined analysis of 12 case control studies nested within prospective cohorts. Gut. 2001;**49**:347-353

[6] de Martel C, Ferlay J, Franceschi S, Vignat J, Bray F, Forman D, Plummer M. Global burden of cancers attributable to infections in 2008: A review and synthetic analysis. Lancet Oncology. 2012;**13**:607-615

[7] O'Connor A, O'Morain CA, Ford AC. Population screening and treatment of Helicobacter pylori infection. Nature Reviews Gastroenterology & Hepatology. 2017;**14**:230-240

[8] Yeh JM, Goldie SJ, Kuntz KM, Ezzati M. Effects of Helicobacter pylori infection and smoking on gastric cancer incidence in China: A population-level analysis of trends and projections. Cancer Causes Control. 2009;**20**:2021-2029

[9] Chiba T, Marusawa H, Seno H, Watanabe N. Mechanism for gastric cancer development by Helicobacter pylori infection. Journal of Gastroenterology and Hepatology. 2008;**23**:1175-1181

[10] Correa P. Human gastric carcinogenesis: A multistep and multifactorial process—First American Cancer Society Award Lecture on Cancer Epidemiology and Prevention. Cancer Research. 1992;**52**:6735-6740

[11] Sheibani S, Mahmoudian RA, Abbaszadegan MR, Chamani J, Memar B, Gholamin M. Expression analysis of matrix metalloproteinase-13 in human gastric cancer in the presence of Helicobacter Pylori infection. Cancer Biomarkers. 2017;**18**(4):349-356

[12] Hanahan D, Weinberg RA. Hallmarks of cancer: The next generation. Cell. 2011;**144**: 646-674

[13] Wu CW, Chi CW, Hsieh MC, Chao MF, Lui WY, P'Eng FK. Serum tumor necrosis factor in patients with gastric cancer. Anticancer Research. 1998;**18**:1597-1599

[14] Bagheri V, Memar B, Momtazi AA, Sahebkar A, Gholamin M, Abbaszadegan MR. Cytokine networks and their association with Helicobacter pylori infection in gastric carcinoma. Journal of Cellular Physiology. 2017;**9999**:1-13

[15] Naumann M, Sokolova O, Tegtmeyer N, Backert S. Helicobacter pylori: A paradigm pathogen for subverting host cell signal transmission. Trends in Microbiology. 2017;**25**:316-328

[16] Epstein MA, Achong BG, Barr YM. Virus particles in cultured lymphoblasts from Burkitt's lymphoma. Lancet. 1964;**1**:702-703

[17] Fukayama M, Hino R, Uozaki H. Epstein–Barr virus and gastric carcinoma: Virus–host interactions leading to carcinoma. Cancer Science. 2008;**99**:1726-1733

[18] Tsang CM, Deng W, Yip YL, Zeng MS, Lo KW, Tsao SW. Epstein-Barr virus infection and persistence in nasopharyngeal epithelial cells. Chinese Journal of Cancer. 2014;**33**:549-555

[19] Tsai MH, Raykova A, Klinke O, Bernhardt K, Gartner K, Leung CS, Geletneky K, Sertel S, Munz C, Feederle R, Delecluse HJ. Spontaneous lytic replication and epitheliotropism define an Epstein-Barr virus strain found in carcinomas. Cell Reports. 2013;**5**:458-470

[20] Abe H, Maeda D, Hino R, Otake Y, Isogai M, Ushiku AS, Matsusaka K, Kunita A, Ushiku T, Uozaki H, Tateishi Y, Hishima T, Iwasaki Y, Ishikawa S, Fukayama M. ARID1A expression loss in gastric cancer: Pathway-dependent roles with and without Epstein-Barr virus infection and microsatellite instability. Virchows Archiv. 2012;**461**:367-377

[21] Abe H, Kaneda A, Fukayama M. Epstein-Barr Virus-Associated gastric carcinoma: Use of host cell machineries and somatic gene mutations. Pathobiology. 2015;**82**:212-223

[22] Chong JM, Sakuma K, Sudo M, Osawa T, Ohara E, Uozaki H, Shibahara J, Kuroiwa K, Tominaga S, Hippo Y, Aburatani H, Funata N, Fukayama M. Interleukin-1beta expression in human gastric carcinoma with Epstein-Barr virus infection. Journal of Virology. 2002;**76**:6825-6831

[23] Fukayama M. Epstein-Barr virus and gastric carcinoma. Pathology International. 2010; **60**:337-350

[24] Cho J, Kang MS, Kim KM. Epstein-Barr Virus-Associated gastric carcinoma and specific features of the accompanying immune response. Journal of Gastric Cancer. 2016;**16**:1-7

[25] D'Elia L, Rossi G, Ippolito R, Cappuccio FP, Strazzullo P. Habitual salt intake and risk of gastric cancer: A meta-analysis of prospective studies. Clinical Nutrition. 2012;**31**:489-498

[26] Tsugane S, Tei Y, Takahashi T, Watanabe S, Sugano K. Salty food intake and risk of Helicobacter pylori infection. Japanese Journal of Cancer Research. 1994;**85**:474-478

[27] Fox JG, Dangler CA, Taylor NS, King A, Koh TJ, Wang TC. High-salt diet induces gastric epithelial hyperplasia and parietal cell loss, and enhances *Helicobacter pylori* colonization in C57BL/6 mice. Cancer Research. 1999;**59**:4823-4828

[28] Camargo MC, Koriyama C, Matsuo K, Kim WH, Herrera-Goepfert R, Liao LM, Yu J, Carrasquilla G, Sung JJ, Alvarado-Cabrero I, Lissowska J, Meneses-Gonzalez F, Yatabe Y, Ding T, Hu N, Taylor PR, Morgan DR, Gulley ML, Torres J, Akiba S, Rabkin CS. Case-case comparison of smoking and alcohol risk associations with Epstein-Barr virus-positive gastric cancer. International Journal of Cancer. 2014;**134**:948-953

[29] Tramacere I, Negri E, Pelucchi C, Bagnardi V, Rota M, Scotti L, Islami F, Corrao G, La Vecchia C, Boffetta P. A meta-analysis on alcohol drinking and gastric cancer risk. Annals of Oncology. 2012;**23**:28-36

[30] Everatt R, Tamosiunas A, Kuzmickiene I, Virviciute D, Radisauskas R, Reklaitiene R, Milinaviciene E. Alcohol consumption and risk of gastric cancer: A cohort study of men in Kaunas, Lithuania, with up to 30 years follow-up. BMC Cancer. 2012;**12**:475

[31] Kelley JR, Duggan JM. Gastric cancer epidemiology and risk factors. Journal of Clinical Epidemiology. 2003;**56**:1-9

[32] Lauren P. The two histological main types of gastric carcinoma: Diffuse and So-Called Intestinal-Type carcinoma. An attempt at a Histo-Clinical classification. Acta Pathologica et Microbiologica Scandinavica. 1965;**64**:31-49

[33] Brunicardi FC, Schwartz SI. Schwartz's Principles of Surgery. 8th ed. New York: McGraw-Hill, Medical Pub. Division; 2005

[34] Nguyen LH, Robinton DA, Seligson MT, Wu L, Li L, Rakheja D, Comerford SA, Ramezani S, Sun X, Parikh MS, Yang EH, Powers JT, Shinoda G, Shah SP, Hammer RE, Daley GQ, Zhu H. Lin28b is sufficient to drive liver cancer and necessary for its maintenance in murine models. Cancer Cell. 2014;**26**:248-261

[35] Finkielstain GP, Forcinito P, Lui JC, Barnes KM, Marino R, Makaroun S, Nguyen V, Lazarus JE, Nilsson O, Baron J. An extensive genetic program occurring during postnatal growth in multiple tissues. Endocrinology. 2009;**150**:1791-1800

[36] The Cancer Genome Atlas Research Network. Comprehensive molecular characterization of gastric adenocarcinoma. Nature. 2014;**513**:202-209

[37] Murphy G, Pfeiffer R, Camargo MC, Rabkin CS. Meta-analysis shows that prevalence of Epstein-Barr virus-positive gastric cancer differs based on sex and anatomic location. Gastroenterology. 2009;**137**:824-833

[38] Matsusaka K, Kaneda A, Nagae G, Ushiku T, Kikuchi Y, Hino R, Uozaki H, Seto Y, Takada K, Aburatani H, Fukayama M. Classification of Epstein-Barr virus-positive gastric cancers by definition of DNA methylation epigenotypes. Cancer Research. 2011;**71**:7187-7197

[39] Toyota M, Ahuja N, Suzuki H, Itoh F, Ohe-Toyota M, Imai K, Baylin SB, Issa JP. Aberrant methylation in gastric cancer associated with the CpG island methylator phenotype. Cancer Research. 1999;**59**:5438-5442

[40] Ridley AJ, Schwartz MA, Burridge K, Firtel RA, Ginsberg MH, Borisy G, Parsons JT, Horwitz AR. Cell migration: Integrating signals from front to back. Science. 2003;**302**: 1704-1709

[41] Thumkeo D, Watanabe S, Narumiya S. Physiological roles of Rho and Rho effectors in mammals. European Journal of Cell Biology. 2013;**92**:303-315

[42] Aznar S, Valeron PF, del Rincon SV, Perez LF, Perona R, Lacal JC. Simultaneous tyrosine and serine phosphorylation of STAT3 transcription factor is involved in Rho A GTPase oncogenic transformation. Molecular Biology of the Cell. 2001;**12**:3282-3294

[43] Yu H, Jove R. The STATs of cancer—New molecular targets come of age. Nature Reviews Cancer. 2004;**4**:97-105

[44] Carthew RW, Sontheimer EJ. Origins and mechanisms of miRNAs and siRNAs. Cell. 2009;**136**:642-655

[45] Lee Y, Han J, Yeom KH, Jin H, Kim VN. Drosha in primary microRNA processing. Cold Spring Harbor Symposia on Quantitative Biology. 2006;**71**:51-57

[46] Han J, Lee Y, Yeom KH, Kim YK, Jin H, Kim VN. The Drosha-DGCR8 complex in primary microRNA processing. Genes & Development. 2004;**18**:3016-3027

[47] Lund E, Guttinger S, Calado A, Dahlberg JE, Kutay U. Nuclear export of microRNA precursors. Science. 2004;**303**:95-98

[48] Bartel DP. MicroRNAs: Genomics, biogenesis, mechanism, and function. Cell. 2004;**116**: 281-297

[49] Miranda KC, Huynh T, Tay Y, Ang YS, Tam WL, Thomson AM, Lim B, Rigoutsos I. A pattern-based method for the identification of MicroRNA binding sites and their corresponding heteroduplexes. Cell. 2006;**126**:1203-1217

[50] Kang W, Tong JH, Lung RW, Dong Y, Zhao J, Liang Q, Zhang L, Pan Y, Yang W, Pang JC, Cheng AS, Yu J, To KF. Targeting of YAP1 by microRNA-15a and microRNA-16-1 exerts tumor suppressor function in gastric adenocarcinoma. Molecular Cancer. 2015;**14**:52

[51] Volinia S, Calin GA, Liu CG, Ambs S, Cimmino A, Petrocca F, Visone R, Iorio M, Roldo C, Ferracin M, Prueitt RL, Yanaihara N, Lanza G, Scarpa A, Vecchione A, Negrini M, Harris CC, Croce CM. A microRNA expression signature of human solid tumors defines cancer gene targets. Proceedings of the National Academy of Sciences of the United States of America. 2006;**103**:2257-2261

[52] Zhang Z, Li Z, Gao C, Chen P, Chen J, Liu W, Xiao S, Lu H. miR-21 plays a pivotal role in gastric cancer pathogenesis and progression. Laboratory Investigation; A Journal of Technical Methods and Pathology. 2008;**88**:1358-1366

[53] Shiotani A, Murao T, Kimura Y, Matsumoto H, Kamada T, Kusunoki H, Inoue K, Uedo N, Iishi H, Haruma K. Identification of serum miRNAs as novel non-invasive biomarkers for detection of high risk for early gastric cancer. British Journal of Cancer. 2013;**109**:2323-2330

[54] Li BS, Zhao YL, Guo G, Li W, Zhu ED, Luo X, Mao XH, Zou QM, Yu PW, Zuo QF, Li N, Tang B, Liu KY, Xiao B. Plasma microRNAs, miR-223, miR-21 and miR-218, as novel potential biomarkers for gastric cancer detection. Plos One. 2012;**7**:e41629

[55] Cui L, Zhang X, Ye G, Zheng T, Song H, Deng H, Xiao B, Xia T, Yu X, Le Y, Guo J. Gastric juice MicroRNAs as potential biomarkers for the screening of gastric cancer. Cancer. 2013;**119**:1618-1626

[56] Wang D, Fan Z, Liu F, Zuo J. Hsa-miR-21 and Hsa-miR-29 in tissue as potential diagnostic and prognostic biomarkers for gastric cancer. Cellular Physiology and Biochemistry: International Journal of Experimental Cellular Physiology, Biochemistry, and Pharmacology. 2015;**37**:1454-1462

[57] Asangani IA, Rasheed SA, Nikolova DA, Leupold JH, Colburn NH, Post S, Allgayer H. MicroRNA-21 (miR-21) post-transcriptionally downregulates tumor suppressor Pdcd4 and stimulates invasion, intravasation and metastasis in colorectal cancer. Oncogene. 2008;**27**:2128-2136

[58] Zhang JG, Wang JJ, Zhao F, Liu Q, Jiang K, Yang GH. MicroRNA-21 (miR-21) represses tumor suppressor PTEN and promotes growth and invasion in non-small cell lung cancer (NSCLC). Clinica Chimica Acta; International Journal of Clinical Chemistry. 2010;**411**:846-852

[59] Orimo A, Gupta PB, Sgroi DC, Arenzana-Seisdedos F, Delaunay T, Naeem R, Carey VJ, Richardson AL, Weinberg RA. Stromal fibroblasts present in invasive human breast carcinomas promote tumor growth and angiogenesis through elevated SDF-1/CXCL12 secretion. Cell. 2005;**121**:335-348

[60] Pietras K, Ostman A. Hallmarks of cancer: Interactions with the tumor stroma. Experimental Cell Research. 2010;**316**:1324-1331

[61] Bhowmick NA, Neilson EG, Moses HL. Stromal fibroblasts in cancer initiation and progression. Nature. 2004;**432**:332-337

[62] Lagace R, Grimaud JA, Schurch W, Seemayer TA. Myofibroblastic stromal reaction in carcinoma of the breast: Variations of collagenous matrix and structural glycoproteins. Virchows Archiv A Pathological Anatomy and Histology. 1985;**408**:49-59

[63] Brown LF, Guidi AJ, Schnitt SJ, Van De Water L, Iruela-Arispe ML, Yeo TK, Tognazzi K, Dvorak HF. Vascular stroma formation in carcinoma in situ, invasive carcinoma, and metastatic carcinoma of the breast. Clinical Cancer Research. 1999;**5**:1041-1056

[64] Hanamura N, Yoshida T, Matsumoto E, Kawarada Y, Sakakura T. Expression of fibronectin and tenascin-C mRNA by myofibroblasts, vascular cells and epithelial cells in human colon adenomas and carcinomas. International Journal of Cancer. 1997;**73**:10-15

[65] Park JE, Lenter MC, Zimmermann RN, Garin-Chesa P, Old LJ, Rettig WJ. Fibroblast activation protein, a dual specificity serine protease expressed in reactive human tumor stromal fibroblasts. Journal of Biological Chemistry. 1999;**274**:36505-36512

[66] DeClerck YA. Interactions between tumour cells and stromal cells and proteolytic modification of the extracellular matrix by metalloproteinases in cancer. European Journal of Cancer. 2000;**36**:1258-1268

[67] Huang WB, Zhou XJ, Chen JY, Zhang LH, Meng K, Ma HH, Lu ZF. CD10-positive stromal cells in gastric carcinoma: Correlation with invasion and metastasis. Japanese Journal of Clinical Oncology. 2005;**35**:245-250

[68] Wu X, Tao P, Zhou Q, Li J, Yu Z, Wang X, Li C, Yan M, Zhu Z, Liu B, Su L. IL-6 secreted by cancer-associated fibroblasts promotes epithelial-mesenchymal transition and metastasis of gastric cancer via JAK2/STAT3 signaling pathway. Oncotarget. 2017;**8**:20741-20750

[69] Landskron G, De la Fuente M, Thuwajit P, Thuwajit C, Hermoso MA. Chronic inflammation and cytokines in the tumor microenvironment. Journal of Immunology Research. 2014;**2014**:149185

[70] Huang L, Wu RL, Xu AM. Epithelial-mesenchymal transition in gastric cancer. American Journal of Translational Research. 2015;**7**:2141-2158

[71] Direkze NC, Hodivala-Dilke K, Jeffery R, Hunt T, Poulsom R, Oukrif D, Alison MR, Wright NA. Bone marrow contribution to tumor-associated myofibroblasts and fibroblasts. Cancer Research. 2004;**64**:8492-8495

[72] Matsumoto T, Kuroda R, Mifune Y, Kawamoto A, Shoji T, Miwa M, Asahara T, Kurosaka M. Circulating endothelial/skeletal progenitor cells for bone regeneration and healing. Bone. 2008;**43**:434-439

[73] Takahashi Y, Cleary KR, Mai M, Kitadai Y, Bucana CD, Ellis LM. Significance of vessel count and vascular endothelial growth factor and its receptor (KDR) in intestinal-type gastric cancer. Clinical Cancer Research. 1996;**2**:1679-1684

[74] Chung HW, Lim JB. Role of the tumor microenvironment in the pathogenesis of gastric carcinoma. World Journal of Gastroenterology. 2014;**20**:1667-1680

[75] Maeda K, Chung YS, Ogawa Y, Takatsuka S, Kang SM, Ogawa M, Sawada T, Sowa M. Prognostic value of vascular endothelial growth factor expression in gastric carcinoma. Cancer. 1996;**77**:858-863

[76] Tanimoto H, Yoshida K, Yokozaki H, Yasui W, Nakayama H, Ito H, Ohama K, Tahara E. Expression of basic fibroblast growth factor in human gastric carcinomas. Virchows Archiv. B, Cell Pathology Including Molecular Pathology. 1991;**61**:263-267

[77] Kasashima H, Yashiro M, Nakamae H, Kitayama K, Masuda G, Kinoshita H, Fukuoka T, Hasegawa T, Nakane T, Hino M, Hirakawa K, Ohira M. CXCL1-Chemokine (C-X-C Motif) receptor 2 signaling stimulates the recruitment of bone Marrow-Derived mesenchymal cells into Diffuse-Type gastric cancer stroma. American Journal of Pathology. 2016;**186**:3028-3039

[78] Huang MM, Guo AB, Sun JF, Chen XL, Yin ZY. Angiotensin II promotes the progression of human gastric cancer. Molecular Medicine Reports. 2014;**9**:1056-1060

[79] Wang L, Zhou R, Zhao Y, Dong S, Zhang J, Luo Y, Huang N, Shi M, Bin J, Liao Y, Liao W. MACC-1 promotes Endothelium-Dependent angiogenesis in gastric cancer by activating TWIST1/VEGF-A signal pathway. PLoS One. 2016;**11**:e0157137

[80] Yancopoulos GD, Davis S, Gale NW, Rudge JS, Wiegand SJ, Holash J. Vascular-specific growth factors and blood vessel formation. Nature. 2000;**407**:242-248

[81] Shah MA, Ramanathan RK, Ilson DH, Levnor A, D'Adamo D, O'Reilly E, Tse A, Trocola R, Schwartz L, Capanu M, Schwartz GK, Kelsen DP. Multicenter phase II study of irinotecan, cisplatin, and bevacizumab in patients with metastatic gastric or gastroesophageal junction adenocarcinoma. Journal of Clinical Oncology. 2006;**24**:5201-5206

[82] Ohtsu A, Shah MA, Van Cutsem E, Rha SY, Sawaki A, Park SR, Lim HY, Yamada Y, Wu J, Langer B, Starnawski M, Kang YK. Bevacizumab in combination with chemotherapy as first-line therapy in advanced gastric cancer: A randomized, double-blind, placebo-controlled phase III study. Journal of Clinical Oncology. 2011;**29**:3968-3976

[83] Shan F, Miao R, Xue K, Li Z, Bu Z, Wu A, Zhang L, Wu X, Zong X, Wang X, Li S, Ji X, Jia Z, Ji J. Controlling angiogenesis in gastric cancer: A systematic review of anti-angiogenic trials. Cancer Letters. 2016;**380**;598-607

[84] Blankenstein T, Coulie PG, Gilboa E, Jaffee EM. The determinants of tumour immunogenicity. Nature Reviews Cancer. 2012;**12**:307-313

[85] Subhash VV, Yeo MS, Tan WL, Yong WP. Strategies and advancements in harnessing the immune system for gastric cancer immunotherapy. Journal of Immunology Research. 2015;**2015**:308574

[86] Zhang WJ, Zhou ZH, Guo M, Yang LQ, Xu YY, Pang TH, Gao ST, Xu XY, Sun Q, Feng M, Wang H, Lu CL, Wu GZ, Guan WX, Xu GF. High infiltration of polarized CD163+ tumor-associated macrophages correlates with aberrant expressions of CSCs markers, and predicts prognosis in patients with recurrent gastric cancer. Journal of Cancer. 2017;**8**:363-370

[87] Kim KJ, Lee KS, Cho HJ, Kim YH, Yang HK, Kim WH, Kang GH. Prognostic implications of tumor-infiltrating FoxP3+ regulatory T cells and CD8+ cytotoxic T cells in microsatellite-unstable gastric cancers. Human Pathology. 2014;**45**:285-293

[88] Liu K, Yang K, Wu B, Chen H, Chen X, Jiang L, Ye F, He D, Lu Z, Xue L, Zhang W, Li Q, Zhou Z, Mo X, Hu J. Tumor-Infiltrating immune cells are associated with prognosis of gastric cancer. Medicine (Baltimore). 2015;**94**:e1631

[89] Mittal D, Gubin MM, Schreiber RD, Smyth MJ. New insights into cancer immunoediting and its three component phases—Elimination, equilibrium and escape. Current Opinion in Immunology. 2014;**27**:16-25

[90] Tumeh PC, Harview CL, Yearley JH, Shintaku IP, Taylor EJ, Robert L, Chmielowski B, Spasic M, Henry G, Ciobanu V, West AN, Carmona M, Kivork C, Seja E, Cherry G, Gutierrez AJ, Grogan TR, Mateus C, Tomasic G, Glaspy JA, Emerson RO, Robins H, Pierce RH, Elashoff DA, Robert C, Ribas A. PD-1 blockade induces responses by inhibiting adaptive immune resistance. Nature. 2014;**515**:568-571

[91] Herbst RS, Soria JC, Kowanetz M, Fine GD, Hamid O, Gordon MS, Sosman JA, McDermott DF, Powderly JD, Gettinger SN, Kohrt HE, Horn L, Lawrence DP, Rost S, Leabman M, Xiao Y, Mokatrin A, Koeppen H, Hegde PS, Mellman I, Chen DS, Hodi FS. Predictive correlates of response to the anti-PD-L1 antibody MPDL3280A in cancer patients. Nature. 2014;**515**:563-567

[92] Zhang M, Dong Y, Liu H, Wang Y, Zhao S, Xuan Q, Zhang Q. The clinicopathological and prognostic significance of PD-L1 expression in gastric cancer: A meta-analysis of 10 studies with 1,901 patients. Scientific Reports. 2016;**6**:37933

Chapter 3

The Purview of Phytotherapy in the Management of Gastric Ulcer

Sabiu Saheed, Ajani Emmanuel Oladipo,
Taofik Olatunde Sunmonu,
Fatai Oladunni Balogun and
Anofi Omotayo Tom Ashafa

Additional information is available at the end of the chapter

http://dx.doi.org/10.5772/intechopen.70007

Abstract

Stomach/gastric ulcer is a debilitating disease affecting more than 10% of the global population. Sufferers often have chronic pains with life-threatening gastrointestinal haemorrhage or perforation. Since the first diagnosis of stomach ulcer (SU) in the 19th century, excessive gastric juice that eroded the mucosa of the stomach was opined as its major cause. Efforts were channelled toward effective control of the resulting acid build-up through the use of antiulcer medications and reduction in stress-induced activities, which may aggravate gastric hyperacidity. An intense treatment option involved vagotomy (surgically severing the nerves surrounding an ulcer) to prevent hyperacidity and further perforation of the stomach epithelium. Despite these interventions, SU disease remained an impediment to clinical practice. Literatures revealed that many botanicals have been used to treat SU and this is hinged on their being endowed with antiulcerogenic phytonutrients of therapeutic significance. In this review, attempts have been made to highlight the main mechanisms of action and limitations of the conventional antiulcerogenic drugs, various antiulcerogenic experimental models, as well as compile selected medicinal plants and their implicated phytonutrients that will ultimately and eventually present effective and globally competitive exciting opportunities for the development of new lead therapeutics for the management of SU disorders.

Keywords: antiulcerogenic, gastric ulcer, gastropathy, hemorrhage, *Helicobacter pylori*, pepsin, perforation, phytonutrients, vagotomy

1. Introduction

Ulcer is an open sore of the biological membrane characterized by sloughing of inflamed dead tissue [1]. More specifically, it could either occur as a lesion on the surface of the skin or a mucous membrane with significant superficial loss of tissue. Although, ulcers may be encountered at almost any part of the body, they are mostly found on the skin of the lower extremities and in the gastrointestinal tract [2]. There are many types of ulcer including mouth, esophageal, peptic and genital ulcer. Of these, peptic ulcer (PU) is the most prevalent [2]. The PUs are erosion of lining of either the stomach or duodenum [3] and this has availed the two most common types of PU as the gastric/stomach ulcer (SU) and duodenal ulcer. A person may have both gastric and duodenal ulcers at the same time. SUs are located in the stomach and mainly characterized by hemorrhage and pain. Other symptoms may include nausea, vomiting, and weight loss. Although patients with SU have normal or diminished acid production, yet ulcers may occur even in complete absence of acid [3]. Generally, pain occurs when the stomach is empty and relieves after eating. In some cases, SU can be life threatening with symptoms like bloody stool, severe abdominal pain, and cramps coupled with blood vomiting [4].

Under normal conditions, a physiologic balance exists between gastric acid secretion and mucosal defense. The epithelial cells of the stomach secrete mucus in response to irritation of the epithelial lining and as a result of cholinergic stimulation [5]. Ordinarily, the superficial portion of the gastric mucosa is jelly-like and impermeable to acid and pepsin. Other gastric cells secrete bicarbonate, which buffers acid that lies penultimate to the mucosa. Also, the prostaglandins of the E (PGE) type of the epithelia offered significant protection by increasing the bicarbonate content and consequently strengthening the mucous layer. However, when the acid and pepsin enters the epithelial cells, further fortifying mechanisms are triggered to ameliorate injury [5]. This may be best observed within the epithelial cells, where ion pumps in the basolateral cell membrane aids intracellular pH regulation through removal of excess H^+ and subsequent migration of healthy cells to the site of injury. By so doing, the acid that diffused through the injured mucosa is effectively removed by the flow of blood in the mucosa. This also provides bicarbonate to the superficial epithelial cells. However, when there is disequilibrium between offensive (acid, pepsin, and *Helicobacter pylori*) and defensive factors (mucin, prostaglandin, bicarbonate, nitric oxide, and growth factors), the pathophysiological features of SU become evident [6]. Although, SU was once believed to be caused by spicy food and stress, they have however been established to be mere aggravating factors while the real causes include reaction to various medications, particularly nonsteroidal anti-inflammatory drugs (NSAIDS) and *H. pylori* infection [7]. *H. pylori*, NSAIDS, emotional stress, alcohol abuse, and smoking are the principal etiological factors associated with SU [8]. Usually, SU occur as breaks across the entire length of the stomach epithelia and in some cases, the deeper layers of the muscle wall are considerably affected. This disruption of the mucosal integrity may potentiate perforation, bleeding, obstruction, pain and death, if proficient treatments are not timely administered. The exclusive production of urease by *H. pylori* renders its microenvironment alkaline and allows its long-lasting survival in the hostile acidic environment of the stomach, where it either worsens the severity of SU disease or merely causes mucosal inflammation. More often in SU cases, inflammation is secondary to the colonizing action of *H. pylori* on the gastric mucosa [5]. In patients infected with *H. pylori*, high levels of gastrin and pepsinogen and reduced levels of somatostatin have been measured [5]. Most patients with SU have impaired gastric bicarbonate secretion, which has also proven to be caused by *H. pylori* because its eradication reverses the defect [9]. Similarly, pepsin (a proteolytic enzyme) and HCl are both essential for food digestion but at the same time have the tendency to erode the cell linings of the digestive system if secreted in excess. Although, the stomach defends itself from these aggravating factors by creating a mucus coating and producing bicarbonates, *H. pylori* infection and NSAIDS can impair the protective functions and make the linings of the gastrointestinal tract susceptible to HCl and pepsin action and consequently results in the formation of ulceration [10].

Globally, SU is the most prevalent gastrointestinal disorder ever known, affecting more than 10% of people and accounting for an estimated 15,000 mortality yearly [11]. The annual incidence of SU perforation and hemorrhage were 3.8–14.0 and 19.4–57.0 per 100,000 persons, respectively and this is anticipated to further worsen if no practical and viable alternatives are sought [12]. Specifically in the United States, PU disease affects approximately 4.5 million people annually and about 10% of the US population has evidence of a SU at some point in their life time [5]. Initially, PU diseases were more prevalent in the male populations but the current statistics suggest quite similar figures in both males and females with the overall lifetime prevalence tending toward 8–11% and 11–14% in women and men, respectively [5]. The age trends for the occurrence of PU show appreciably declining rates in younger males, while it is increasing steadily in older women. The statistics for SU disease in other countries is variable and is hinged primarily on the major causes of the disease: *H. pylori* and NSAIDs [13].

Although, orthodox medicine has provided succor in the management of SU disease over the years, a significant percentage of the global population still use traditional systems of medicine to manage and treat SU due to better cultural acceptability, improved compatibility, affordability, and lesser side effects [14]. The present study was conducted to review medicinal plants considered as gastroprotective and healing agents on SUs with particular focus on selected antiulcerogenic botanicals and their implicated phytonutrients. To achieve this, information were retrieved from online databases (Google, Pubmed, MEDLINE, Science Direct, Scopus and SID) in form of published articles, books, conference proceedings and other high profile intellectual resources. The retrieved studies either showed effectiveness of these plants or indirectly their efficacy on the involved mechanisms in the treatment of SU.

2. The conventional therapy for stomach ulcer management

SU therapy has witnessed many strides over the last decades and a number of drugs are now available for its treatment. Since the occurrence of SU disease is attributable to either pepsin action and hyperacidity or inadequate mucosal resistance, hence, its effective management lies exclusively in stemming the aggressive factors or fortify the defensive mechanisms. A corner stone in this approach was the advent of histamine H_2-receptors and the respective antagonist [15], which signified a landmark achievement in the management of disorders characterized by gastric hypersecretion. The H_2-antagonists were instantaneously identified as potent and safe agents which may replace the previously used drugs. For instance, the appearance of cimetidine (an H_2-antagonist agent), led to the virtual disappearance of drugs of unknown mechanism like gefarnate, sulphoglycopeptide, amilopectine, zolimidine, xylamide, etc. Despite the inherent improvement witnessed with the use of the H_2-antagonist over the previously used drugs, their untoward reactions have undermined their appreciable application. Generally, the antiulcer drugs may be classified according to the site and/or mechanism of action as: (a) antacids; (b) gastric muscle stimulants; (c) agents which protect the mucosa, increase mucosal resistance or coat ulcer craters; (d) antisecretory drugs, which may be anticholinergic agents; (e) corticohypothalamic drugs; and (f) proton pump inhibitors.

2.1. Antacids

It is noteworthy that either antacid mixtures or combinations of antacids with other compounds are more commonly used than single-entity antacids [15]. These kinds of formulation have been made to elicit a better neutralizing effect and to extenuate side effects associated with single constituent entities. The calcium and aluminium combinations reduce diarrhea while magnesium caters well for constipation. Similarly, a combination of slow- and fast-acting agents could increase the total buffering time. More improved benefits are claimed for mixtures having alginic acid (a foam-forming agent), which floats above the gastric juice with eventual aiding of contact between the antacid and the mucosa. In the event of gastroesophageal reflux, the alginic acid appears to prevent reflux by being the first to come in contact with the esophagus. By so doing, further erosion by the gastric acid is effectively prevented. Also, when simethicone (dimethylpolysiloxanes with characteristics antifoaming and water-repellant properties) is used, defoaming the gastric juice to reduce flatulence and gastroesophageal reflux is achieved. However, the resulting contributory adverse effects of the respective constituent in the antacid especially gastric irritation are a major challenge consistent with the use of antacids.

2.2. Gastric muscle stimulants

In individuals with stomach atony where there is consequential prolonged contact time between acid and mucosa due to the delay in gastric emptying, stimulants of gastric motility produce satisfactory outcomes. Domperidone and metoclopramide are the two most widely used compounds in this category. While both accelerates gastric emptying in experimental animals and humans, the metoclopramide still acts via other four important mechanisms that have made it more potent: (i) a cholinergic effect on muscarinic receptors; (ii) a direct effect on smooth muscle; (iii) an effect on specific centers regulating gastrointestinal motility; and (iv) a release of motilin which could be strongly responsible for the effects on the proximal bowel [15].

2.3. Mucosa protecting agents

Compounds like sucralfate, carbenoxolone and chelated bismuthate belong to this class of drugs. The sucralfate (a complex of sucrose and aluminium hydroxide) potentiates its action by inhibiting gastric hydrolysis with significant affinity for ulcerated mucosa. It forms a complex with susceptible proteins (fibrinogen, albumin etc) that adhere to the ulcerated area, thereby shielding against acid, pepsin action and penetration of bile acid. The merits of sucralfate over other antiulcer drugs relate to a lack of systemic effect due to the poor absorption of the compound [16]. The disadvantages include a certain delay in gastric emptying and constipation which affects almost 2% of the sufferers. Furthermore, compliance is another issue of concern as sucralfate must be taken four times daily (q.i.d.) and at least one hour before meals to be optimally effective. While chelated bismuthate and carbenoxolone works quite similar to sucralfate, appreciable incidence of aldosterone-like adverse effects (sodium and fluid retention, hypertension etc) have hampered their use.

2.4. Drugs with antisecretory effect

2.4.1. Anticholinergics

Despite that the drugs in this class have been used for many years, information on their ulcer healing capacity is still elusive. This may be attributable to the radiological method that was initially used but later found not to be very effective in wound healing assessment. Hyoscyamine, atropine, phentonium, propantheline and methantheline with characteristic ganglion-blocking and antimuscarinic effects are the classical examples of anticholinergics. Subsequent to the discovery and acceptance of the H_2-antagonists, the anticholinergics virtually disappeared due to inherent adverse effects of dry mouth, blurring of vision, delay in gastric emptying, tachycardia, possible constipation, and urinary retention.

2.4.2. H_2-antagonists

Undoubtedly, the H_2-antagonists are the most significant agents for the management and treatment of SU and for pathological conditions characterized by hyperacidity. Burimamide (the prototype of H_2-antagonists) was faced-out because of low oral activity and toxicological concerns. Similarly, metiamide (the 2nd agent in the series), was orally active but potentiated significant bone marrow toxicity in clinical trials. Cimetidine (still the most widely used antiulcer drug), is the 3rd drug in this class and well over 70 million sufferers have so far benefitted from its pharmacological efficacy till date. This was closely followed by ranitidine, which was the first agent with an alkyl furan ring, which substituted the imidazole ring of the preceding H_2- antagonists. More recent reports however suggest that optimum H_2-antagonism may also be achieved also with other different agents. For this class of drugs, not only could potency and efficacy be optimized, the pharmacokinetics could also be modified with the known duration of action of 4–6 h, exclusive to the 'short-acting' H_2-blockers [17], optimized to and beyond 24–48 h to have 'long-acting' H_2-blockers. Generally, over the last three decades, the most frequently used H_2-antagonists in clinical practice are cimetidine, ranitidine and famotidine [2]. However, many adverse reactions such as effects on the endocrine, cardiovascular and central nervous systems (CNS) have been associated with these drugs.

2.5. Corticohypothalamic drugs

A role has been established for the CNS in the regulation of gastric secretion and in the pathogenesis of peptic ulcer, although clarification is required in many areas. It is not surprising that drugs which act specifically on the CNS may exert a beneficial effect on SU, which sometimes is significantly better than other drugs. Trimipramine is a tricyclic antidepressant which causes a slight decrease in gastric secretion that is apparently not connected with its anticholinergic action. Like other traditional tricyclic antidepressants, it may have some H_2-antagonistic effects and may also act on α-adrenoceptors enhancing catecholamine availability at central synapses [18], or may depress central vagal function. However the use of trimipramine in non-depressed ulcer patients is questionable.

2.6. Proton pump inhibitors (PPIs)

At present, PPIs are the most commonly prescribed class of antiulcer drugs. Their mode of action involves blockage of the site of gastric acid secretion in the parietal cell of the stomach [19]. However, because the parietal cells are constantly reproducing in millions, effective inhibition of gastric acid secretion is almost unachievable and this partly explains their relative safety compared to other groups of antiulcer drugs. In general, the incidence of short-term adverse effects subsequent to PPI usage is relatively low and this may be the reason for their being well tolerated. Their long-term use has not been frequently studied and the dearth of information in this regards has made it difficult to make definitive statements [20]. For all the PPIs (omeprazole, lansoprazole, dexlanprazole, esomeprazole, pantoprazole, rabeprazole and ilaprazole), the occurrence of adverse effects are similar, though they have been reported more frequently with omeprazole. This may be due to its longer availability. The common adverse effects with PPIs include headache, nausea, diarrhea, abdominal pain, fatigue and dizziness. Infrequent adverse effects may also include rash, itch, flatulence, constipation, anxiety, depression, myopathies and rhabdomyolysis [21].

3. Ulcer inducing agents/models

The pathological mechanisms of SU disease that compromises its functional capability and the structural integrity has been established to arise mainly through either production of too much acid and pepsin, or weakening of the gastric epithelia that consequently results in too little mucosal resistance [2]. **Table 1** shows some of the known ulcerogenic agents/models and the pathological mechanism involved in their ulcer pathogenesis. A good understanding of the pathogenic mechanism of action of these models is crucial to spotting and either managing or preventing ulceration and the associated disorders.

Agent/model	Underlying mechanism	Reference(s)
NSAIDs (aspirin, indomethacin and ibuprofen)	Gastric acid secretion and inhibition of prostaglandin synthetase activity	[22]
Water-immersion/cold-restraint stress	Release of histamine resulting in increased acid secretion, decreased mucus production and poor flow of gastric blood	[23, 24]
Ethanol	Solubilizes mucous membrane and renders it vulnerable to the proteolytic and hydrolytic actions of HCl and pepsin	[25]
Acetic acid	Induces round, deep ulcers in the stomach through over production of acid secretion	[26]
Histamine	Acid stimulating and vasodilating effect that results to increased vascular permeability of the gastric mucosa	[27]
Reserpine	Degranulation of gastric mast cells consequent to histamine liberation that is facilitated by cholinergic system	[28]
Serotonin	Causes vasoconstriction thereby reducing gastric mucosal blood flow resulting to acute mucosal injury	[29]
Pylorous-ligation	Accumulation of gastric acid that consequently produces ulcer subsequent to the breakdown of gastric mucosal barriers	[30]
Ischemia-reperfusion	Causes erosion of the gastric epithelia due to free radicals formation	[31]
Acetic acid-*H. pylori*	Increased acid secretion and decreased mucus production	[32]
Iron-ascorbic acid	Linked with lipid peroxidation mediated by oxygen radicals	[33]

Table 1. Commonly used experimental models for ulcer induction.

4. Some scientifically validated antiulcerogenic medicinal plants

Despite the rapidly changing concept of SU disease management from conventional vagotomy, H_2-receptor antagonists and antacids to proton pump inhibitors, gastrointestinal toxicity and other inherent adverse effects remain significant impediments to their application in clinical practice. Investigation on the phytotherapeutic applications of medicinal plants that are highly valued and widely used in the traditional systems of medicine have been and still providing efficient formulation for better management of SU [2, 22].

The under-listed medicinal plants have been pharmacological reported to possess antiulcer activity as previously compiled [34–39]. They are:

Acacia arabica (Family: Mimosaceae); *Abutilon indicum* L. (Family: Malvaceae); *Adansonia digitate; Aegle marmelos* (Family: Rutaceae); *Allium sativum* (Family: Liliaceae); *Allophylus serratus* Kurz (Family: Sapindaceae); *Aloe vera* (Family: Liliaceae); *Alstonia scholaris; Annona squamosa* (Family: Annonaceae); *Asparagus racemosus; Azadirachta indica* (Family: Meliaceae); *Bacopa monnieri; Benincasa hispida; Bauhinia purpurea* (Family: Leguminosae); *Bauhinia variegate* (Family: Caesalpiniaceae); *Berberis aristata; Beta vulgaris; Buchanania lanzan* Spreng. (Family:

Anacardiaceae); *Butea frondosa* Roxb. (Family: Fabaceae); *Boswellia serrata* (Family: Burseraceae); *Careya arborea* (Family: Myrtaceae); *Carica papaya* (Family: Caricaceae); *Capsicum annuum* L. (Family: Solanaceae); *Centella asiatica; Cissus quadrangularis* L. (Family: Vitaceae); *Curcuma longa* L. (Family: Zingiberaceae); *Desmostachya bipinnata* (L.) Stapf (Family: Gramineae); *Desmodium gangeticum; Emblica officinalis* (Family: Euphorbiaceae); *Excoecaria agallocha* (Family: Euphorbiaceae); *Garcinia cambogia; Glycyrrhiza glabra* (Family: Leguminosae); *Ficus arnottiana; Ficus religiosa* (Family: Urticaceae); *Hemidesmus indicus; Hibiscus rosa sinensis* (Family: Malvaceae); *Ipomoea batatas* L. (Family: Convolvulaceae); *Ixora pavetta* (Family: Rubiaceae); *Kielmeyera coriacea* Mart (Family: Guttiferae); *Lagenaria siceraria* (Family: Cucurbitaceae); *Leucas lavandulifolia* Sm. (Family: Labiatae); *Mangifera indica* (Family: Anacardiaceae); *Mimosa pudica* (Family: Fabaceae); *Mentha arvensis* L. (Family: Lamiaceaea); *Momordica charantia* (Family: Cucurbitaceae); *Momordica cymbalaria* Hook. (Family: Cucurbitaceae); *Morinda citrifolia; Moringa oleifera* (Family: Moringaceae); *Musa sapientum; Myrtus communis* (Family: Myrtaceae); *Ocimum sanctum* (Family: Lamiaceae); *Oryza sativa* (Family: Gramineae); *Phyllanthus niruri* (Family: Euphorbiaceae); *Plectranthus amboinicus; Polyalthia longifolia* (Family: Annonaceae); *Psidium guyava* (Family: Myrtaceae); *Rhus coriaria* (Family: Anacardiaceae); *Rhizophora mangle* L. (Family: Rhizophoraceae); *Sapindus trifoliatus* L. (Family: Sapindaceae); *Sesbania grandiflora* (Fabaceae); *Shorea robusta* (Family: Dipterocarpaceae); *Solanum nigrum* (Family: Solanaceae); *Tamarindus indica* (Family: Caesalpiniaceae); *Tamarindus indica* (Family: Caesalpiniaceae); *Tecomaria capensis* (Family: Bignoniaceae); *Terminalia chebula* (Family: Combretaceae); *Terminalia pallida; Utleria salicifolia Bedd.* Ex.Hook. F. (Family: Periplocaceae); *Vinca minor* L. (Family: Apocynaceae). A comprehensive list of some selected plants being embraced as antiulcerogenic agents is presented in **Table 2**.

Plant	Family	Plant used	Phytonutrients	Reference(s)
Acacia arabica	Mimosaceae	Gum, leaves	Arabic acid, malate, sugar, mineral elements, tannins	[40, 41]
Achyranthus aspera	Amaranthaseae	Root, seeds	Saponin, glycosides	[42]
Adansonia digitata	Malvaceae	Leaves	Mucilage, glucose, albuminoids, adansonin, tannin	[43]
Aegle marmelos	Rutaceae	Leaves	Flavonoid, tannins, saponin	[44]
Aleo vera	Liliaceae	Whole plant	Aloin, isobarbaloin, emodin, saponin	[45]
Alhagi maurorum	Fabaceae	Root	Terpenes, saponin, tannins	[46]
Allium sativum	Liliaceae	Bulb	Mucilage, starch, albumen, vitamins, sugar, allicin, alliin	[47]
Annona squamosa	Annonaceae	Leaves	Alkaloids, flavonoids, saponini, tannins	[48]
Azadirachta indica	Meliaceae	Leaves	Saponin, flavonoids, phenolics, tannin	[49]
Bauhinia variegate	Caesalpiniaceae	Stem-bark, root	Rutin, quercetin, apigenin, tannin	[50]
Berberis aristata	Berberidaceae	Root	Alkaloids	[51]
Bata vulgaris	Chenopodiaceae	Root	Betin	[52]
Carica papaya	Caricaceae	Fruit, seeds	Papain, pectin, carpaine, carposide	[53]

Plant	Family	Plant used	Phytonutrients	Reference(s)
Centella asiatica	Apiaceae	Whole plant	Flavonoids, narigin, alkaloids, saponin, asiatic acid	[54]
Cordial myxa		Fruit	Tannins, carbohydrate, saponin	[55]
Ficus exasperata	Moraceae	Leaves, stem-bark	Flavonoids, saponin, alkaloids, glycosides, tannins	[2]
Ficus religiosa	Urticaceae	Stem-bark	Tannins, wax, cochtone	[56]
Gossypium barbadense	Malvaceae	Leaves	Gossypol, saponin, steroids, cardiac glycosides	[22]
Gossypium herbaceous	Malvaceae	Flowers	Flavonoids, phenolics, saponin	[57]
Hibiscus rosa sinensis	Malvaceae	Root	Phenolics, cyanidin, hydrocitrate	[58]
Langeneria breviflora	Cucurbitaceae	Fruit, leaves	Saponin, phenolics, cucurbitacin	[59]
Langeneria siceraria	Cucurbitaceae	Fruit	Flavonoids, steroids, phenols, saponin	[42]
Mangifera indica	Anacardiaceae	Leaves	Alkaloids, sterols, saponin, tannins, flavonoids, mangiferin	[60]
Momordica tuberose	Cucurbitaceae	Tubers	Alkaloids, tannins, saponin	[61]
Moringa oleifera	Moringaceae	Leaves	Quercetin, β-sitoterol, β-carotene, alkaloids, tannins, saponin	[62]
Musa paradisiacal	Musaceae	Root, leaves, trunk	Tannins, starch, vitamin C, albuminoids	[42]
Myrtus communis	Myrtaceae	Leaves	Resin, tannins, citrate, malate, sugar	[63]
Nerium indicum	Apocynaceae	Flowers	Alkaloids, glycosides, flavonoids, phenolics, tannins	[64]
Ocimum sanctum	Lamiaceae	Leaves	Alkaloids, tannins, saponin, flavonoids, sterols	[65]
Oryza sativa	Gramineae	Grain, bran	Starch, mineral matter, protein	[66]
Phyllanthus niruri	Euphorbiaceae	Whole plant	Alkaloids, tannins, flavonoids, carbohydrate, glycosides	[67]
Prunus amygdalus	Rosaceae	Seeds, fruit	Ursolic acid, quercetin, flavonoids	[42]
Psidium guyava	Myrtaceae	Leaves, stem-bark	Resin, tannins, cellulose, flavonoids, quercetin, quajaverin	[68]
Rhus coriaria	Anacardiaceae	Whole plant	Tannins, flavonoids	[69]
Sesbania grandiflora	Fabaceae	Leaves	Saponin, tannins, triterpenes	[70]
Smilax china	Smilacaceae	Root	Tannins, resin, saponin, flavonoids	[71]
Solanum nigrum	Solanaceae	Leaves	Flavonoids, saponin, alkaloids, phytosterols	[72]
Spondias mombin	Anacardiaceae	Leaves	Tannins, saponin, flavonoids, phenolics, glycosides	[73]
Tamarindus indica	Caesalpiniaceae	Leaves, seeds	Albuminoids, fiber, pectin, tannins	[74]
Terminalia chebula	Combretaceae	Leaves	Gallic acid, sorbitol, tannins, mucilage	[75]

Table 2. Some selected medicinal plants with antiulcerogenic properties.

Following the experimental demonstration that many medicinal plants are endowed with good antiulcerogenic activity with relatively lesser adverse effect compared with the conventional drugs, further steps have been taken in presenting a good number of them for clinical trials. Despite this giant stride, not many of the medicinal plants have passed market entry stage. To the best of our knowledge, of the many presented for developmental evaluations in 2004, only *Azadirachta indica* (Family: Meliaceae) received remarkable attention at its advance stage of clinical trial. It exhibited significant therapeutic potency by reducing gastric hypersecretion, gastroesophageal and gastroduodenal ulcers [76].

5. Phytonutrients associated with antiulcerogenic activity

Several phytonutrients have proven health benefits and have been reported to elicit significant antiulcerogenic potential in both humans and experimental animal models [73]. While steroid glycosides, tannins, terpenoids and flavonoids have been shown to preserve gastric mucosal against oxidative insults of reactive metabolites and oxidative stress [22, 59], the tendency of phenolic compounds and alkaloids to regulate gastric acid secretion and protect the gastric mucosal epithelia against erosion and other aggressive factors in different ulcer models have been demonstrated [77]. While **Table 1** also presents some of these phytonutrients as being responsible for the elicited antiulcerogenic properties of the plants, several others have also been identified and isolated from diverse plants. Some of these include; saponins, phobaphenes, glucose, luvangetin, tartarate, potash, nimbidin, quercetin, apigenin, papain, chymopapain, pectin, carposide, carotenoids, antheraxanthin, carpaine, resin, euphorbon, caoutchouc, rutin, anthocyanins, cyanindin, kaempferol, sterols, mucilage, terpenoids, kaepferom, ash, starch, fats, proteins, glycosides, ellagic acid, beta sitosterol, gallic acid, limonene, pinene, albuminous matter, cellulose, chlorophyll, mineral salts, myricitin, triterpenes, and sorbitol [37]. These compounds have either been elucidated to decrease acid/pepsin secretion or confer cytoprotection via effective modulation on mucosal defensive factors.

6. Some selected medicinal plants with antiulcerogenic properties in Nigeria

In Nigeria, SU remains a significant public health challenge affecting people of all ages. While its management through orthodox medicine has recorded substantial successes over the years, a considerable proportion of the populace still rely exclusively on complementary and alternative medicine (CAM) in seeking aid to treat and manage SU. This may be due to the ease of accessibility, affordability and minimal side effect associated with the use of medicinal plants [22]. A compilation of selected antiulcerogenic medicinal plants in Nigeria revealed that the most widely used plants in the management of SU are *Occimum basillicum, M. paradisiaca, Aloe vera, Azadiracter indica, Brassica oleracae* and *Carica papaya* [78]. Others include but not limited to the following: *Diodia sarmentosa, Cassia nigricans, Ficus exasperate, Synclisia scabrida, Artocarpus heterophyllus* Lam., *Blighia sapida* Konig., *Dialium guineense* Willd., *Emblica officinalis* Gaertn., *Gongronema latifolium, Ageratum conyzoides, Aloe vera, Artocarpusaltilis, Aspilia africana, Bryophyllum pinnatum, Fluerya aestuans, Musa paradiasiaca, Musa sapientum, Persea Americana, Talinum triangulare, Fluerya aetuans, Brassica oleracae, Acacia nilotica* L., *Alchornea cordifolia Schum & thonn, Anacardium occidentale* L., *Balanites aegyptiaca* L., *Bridelia ferruginea* Benth, *Carica papaya* Linn, *Ficus thonningii* Blume, *Guiera senegalensis* J. F. Gmel, *Hibiscus sabdariffa* L., *Mangifera indica* L., *Momordica charantia* L., *Ocimum gratissium* L., *Piliostigma reticulatum* (DC) Hochst, *Pisidium guajava* L., *Scoparia dulcis, Vernonia kotschyana* Sch. Bip., *Zingiber officinale* Rosc [79].

7. The role of medicinal plants in oxidative gastropathy

Reactive oxygen species (ROS) are a by-product of normal metabolism and have roles in cell signaling and homeostasis [80]. Mechanisms exist that regulate cellular levels of ROS, as their reactive nature may otherwise cause damage to key cellular components including DNA, protein, and lipids [81]. A good number of NSAIDS have been implicated in cellular toxicity leading to oxidative gastropathy [82]. Despite the use of NSAIDS as antipyretic and anti-inflammation agents, and in the treatment of rheumatic, musculoskeletal, and cardiovascular diseases [83], gastrointestinal toxicity through ROS formation has limited their application [84, 85]. It has been proposed that NSAID-mediated gastrointestinal lesions involve the uncoupling of oxidative phosphorylation and inhibition of electron transport chain causing incomplete reduction of oxygen [82]. This they do by tenaciously binding to a site near complex I and ubiquinone, thus facilitating events leading to ROS generation [86, 87]. Subsequently, when the gastric antioxidant capacity is overwhelmed, the epithelia mitochondrial aconitase is inhibited, resulting in the release of iron that reacts with H_2O_2, producing hydroxyl radical. These cascades of event amplify gastric oxidative stress whose consequential effect is manifested as gastropathy [88]. Oxidative stress-induced functional loss is well correlated with numerous disease states including cardiovascular, neurological, cancer, aging processes and gastropathy [83] and is also implicated in a variety of drug-induced toxicities such as SU [2]. Antioxidative and free radical scavenging mechanisms play an important role in the protection against ROS mediated toxicities [89]. Over the past decades, interests in medicinal plants, especially the antioxidative ones, have increased appreciably and they have been elucidated to significantly either protect against or ameliorate ROS-mediated oxidative gastropathy [22, 90]. Such annihilation of ROS in SU diseases have been achieved through induction of enzymic antioxidants (superoxide dismutase, catalase, glutathione reductase and peroxidase) and optimization of reduced glutathione (GSH) contents [2, 22, 59]. Harmonizing the foregoing, a probable mechanism of antioxidative and gastroprotective activities of medicinal plants may be idealized as illustrated in **Figure 1**. This ultimately involves induction and optimization of preventive (catalase, glutathione peroxidase) and chain-breaking (superoxide dismutase, glutathione reductase) antioxidants that subsequently improve gastric GSH level, annihilate liberated reactive metabolite and effectively scavenge ROS (O_2^-, OH^-) (**Figure 1**). This may also be opined to regulate mucosal fluidity and strengthens defensive mechanisms against oxidative gastric damage.

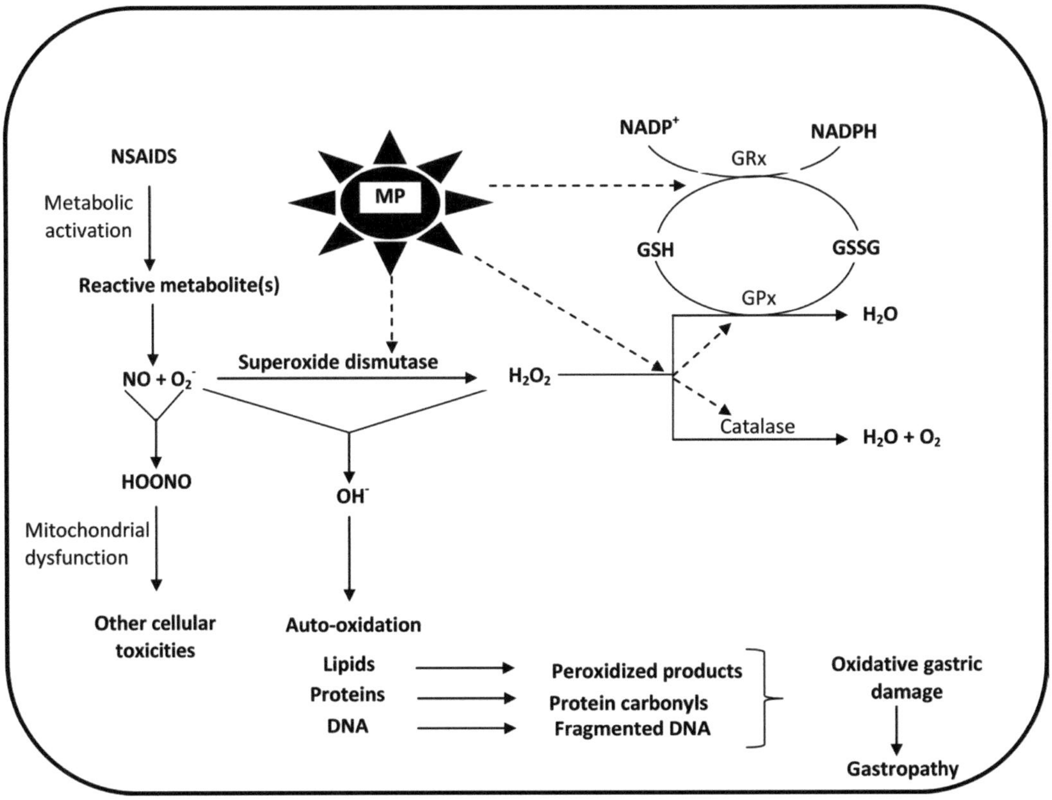

Figure 1. Probable mechanism of antioxidative and gastroprotective capabilities of medicinal plants. The dotted arrows represent sites of induction and optimization by the plants that consequently promote scavenging of O_2^- and OH^-. This will normalize and increase gastric reduced glutathione (GSH) content and promotes its mobilization toward detoxification of the liberated reactive metabolites. NSAIDS, nonsteroidal anti-inflammatory drugs; MP, medicinal plants; GPx, glutathione peroxidase; GRx, glutathione reductase; GSSG, oxidized glutathione.

8. Conclusion

Globally, SU is a devastating disease posing serious threat to the quality of life of humans. It affects significant proportion of the populace in both developed and developing countries. Although, conventional drugs have been used to manage and treat SU sufferers, affordability and inherent side effects have limited their application. Consequently, alternatives are being sought in medicinal plants, which provide a potential source of antiulcerogenic drugs and are widely used in traditional systems of medicine. Several medicinal plants have been investigated for their proven health benefits in SU management with their phytonutrients playing significant roles. Of the phytonutrients, tannins seem to top the list and has suggested probable focus on their characterization for antiulcer therapy. In spite of the impressive experimental evaluation of medicinal plants for the treatment of SU, very few have reached clinical trials and not very many have been marketed. This indicates that the intended benefits of CAM research are not yet having far-reaching effect. Nevertheless, the continuous search for antiulcerogenic agents of plant origin (available as gifts of nature) is imperative. This will ultimately and eventually present effective and globally competitive exciting opportunities for the development of new lead therapeutics for SU and other related disorders.

Author details

Sabiu Saheed[1,2,3]*, Ajani Emmanuel Oladipo[1], Taofik Olatunde Sunmonu[4], Fatai Oladunni Balogun[2] and Anofi Omotayo Tom Ashafa[2]

*Address all correspondence to: saeed.sabiu@gmail.com

1 Phytomedicine, Food Factors and Toxicology Research Laboratory, Biochemistry Department, School of Basic Medical Sciences, Kwara State University, Ilorin, Nigeria

2 Phytomedicine and Phytopharmacology Research Group, Plant Sciences Department, University of the Free State, Phuthaditjhaba, South Africa

3 Department of Microbial, Biochemical, and Food Biotechnology, University of the Free State, Bloemfontein, South Africa

4 Phytomedicine and Plant Biochemistry Research Laboratory, Biochemistry Unit, Department of Biological Sciences, Al-Hikmah University, Ilorin, Nigeria

References

[1] Chan FKL, Graham DY. Review article: prevention of non-steroidal anti-inflammatory drug gastrointestinal complications—Review and recommendations based on risk assessment. Alimentary Pharmacology and Therapeutics. 2004;**19**(10):1051-1061

[2] Sabiu S, Sulyman AO, Garuba T, Sunmonu TO, Abdulrahaman AA. Combined administration of *Spondias mombin* and ficus exasperata leaf extracts stall indomethacin-mediated gastric mucosal onslaught in rats. African Journal of Traditional Complementary Alternative Medicine. 2015;**12**:45-51

[3] Debjit B, Chiranjib C, Tripathi KK, Pankaj J, Sampath KP. Recent trends of treatment and medication peptic ulcerative disorder. International Journal of PharmTech Research. 2010;**2**(1):970-980

[4] Vyawahare NS, Deshmukh VV, Godkari MR, Kagathara VG. Plants with anti-ulcer activity. Pharmacognosy Review. 2009;**3**:108-115

[5] Anand BS. Peptic ulcer diseases. Gastroenterology. 2017;**1**:23-35

[6] Hoogerwerf WA, Pasricha PJ. Agents Used for Control of Gastric Acidity and Treatment of Peptic Ulcers and Gastro Esophageal Reflux Disease, 10th ed. New York, NY, USA: McGraw-Hill; 2001. pp. 1005-1019

[7] Marshall BJ, Warren JR. Unidentified curved bacilli in the stomach of patients with gastritis and peptic ulceration. The Lancet. 1984;**1**(8390):1311-1315

[8] Malfertheiner P, Chan FK, McColl KE. Peptic ulcer disease. The Lancet. 2009;**374**(9699): 1449-1461

[9] Sung JJ, Tsoi KK, Ma YK, Yung MY, Lau JY, Chiu PW. Causes of mortality in patients with peptic ulcer diseases: A prospective cohort study of 10428 cases. American Journal of Gastroenterology. 2010;**105**(1):84-89

[10] Bansal, et al. Herbal approach to peptic ulcer disease: Review. Journal of Bioscience Technology. 2009;**1**:52-58

[11] Shristi B, Neha J, Indu BP, Rajesh G. A review on some Indian medicinal plants for antiulcer activity. Journal of Science Research and Pharmacy. 2012;**1**:6-9

[12] Lau JY, Sung J, Hill C, Henderson C, Howden CW, Metz DC. Systematic review of the epidemiology of complicated peptic ulcer disease: Incidence, recurrence, risk factors and mortality. Digestion. 2011;**84**(2):102-113

[13] Cai S, Garcia RLA, Masso-Gonzalez EL, Hernande-Diaz S. Uncomplicated peptic ulcer disease in the United Kingdom: Trends from 1997 to 2005. Alimentary Pharmacology Therapeutics. 2009;**30**(10):1039-1048

[14] Kumar R. A review on medicinal plants for peptic ulcer. Der Pharmacia Lettre. 2011; **3**(3):414-420

[15] Bertaccini G, Coruzzi G. Pharmacology of the treatment of peptic ulcer disease. Digestive Diseases and Sciences. 1985;**30**(11):43s-51s

[16] Martin F, Farley A, Gagnon M, Bensemana D. Comparison of healing capacities of sucralfate and cimetidine in short treatment of duodenal ulcer. Double blind randomized trial. Gastroenterology. 1982;**82**:401-405

[17] Buyniski JP, Cavanagh RL, Pircio AW, Agieri AA, Crenshaw RR. In: Melchiorre C, Gianella M, editors. Highlights in Receptor Chemistry. Amsterdam: Elsevier; 1984. pp. 195-213

[18] Pendleton RG, McCafferty JP, Roesler JM, Hieble JP. Mechanism for gastric antisecretory effects of desmethylimipramine in rats. European Journal of Pharmacology. 1981;**75**:171-178

[19] Sachar H, Vaidya K, Laine L. Intermittent vs continuous proton pump inhibitor therapy for high-risk bleeding ulcers: a systematic review and meta-analysis. JAMA Internal Medicine. 2014;**174**(11):1755-1762

[20] Corleto VD. Proton pump inhibitor therapy and potential long-term harm. Current Opinion in Endocrinology, Diabetes and Obesity. 2016;**21**(1):3-8

[21] Rossi S, editor. Australian Medicines Handbook 2006. Adelaide: Australian Medicines Handbook 2006

[22] Sabiu S, Ajani EO, Ajao AA, Sunmonu TO, Ibraheem AS, Ibrahim R, Mustapha H, Adekeye AO. Biomembrane stabilization and antiulcerogenic properties of aqueous leaf extract of *Gossypium barbadense* L. (Malvaceae). Beni-Suef University Journal of Basic and Applied Sciences. 2017. http://dx.doi.org/10.1016/j.bjbas.2017.05.007

[23] Senay EC, Levine RJ. Synergism between cold and restraint for rapid production of stress ulcers in rats. Proceedings of the Society for Experimental Biology and Medicine. 1967;**124**(4):1221-1223

[24] Kitagawa H, Fujiwara M, Osumi Y. Effects of water immersion stress on gastric secretion and mucosal blood flow in rats. Gastroenterology. 1979;**77**(2):298-302

[25] Oates PJ, Hakkinen JP. Studies on the mechanism of ethanol-induced gastric damage in rats. Gastroenterology. 1988;**94**(1):10-21

[26] Okabe S, Amagase K. An overview of acetic acid ulcer models: The history and state of the art of peptic ulcer research. Biological and Pharmaceutical Bulletin. 2005;**28**(8):1321-1341

[27] Cho CH, Pfeiffer CJ. Gastrointestinal ulceration in the guinea pig in response to dimaprit, histamine, and H_1- and H_2-blocking agents. Digestive Diseases and Sciences. 1981;**26**(4):306-311

[28] Singh S. Evaluation of gastric anti-ulcer activity of fixed oil of *Ocimum basilicum Linn*. and its possible mechanism of action. Indian Journal of Experimental Biology. 1999;**37**(3):253-257

[29] LePard KJ, Stephens RL. Serotonin inhibits gastric acid secretion through a 5-hydroxy-tryptamine1-like receptor in the rat. Journal of Pharmacology and Experimental Therapeutics. 1994;**270**(3):1139-1147

[30] Shay H, Komarov SA, Fels SS, Meranze D, Gruenstein M, Siplet H. A simple method for the uniform production of gastric ulceration in the rat, Gastroenterology. 1945;**5**:43-61

[31] Wada K, Kamisaki Y, Kitano M, Kishimoto Y, Nakamoto K, Itoh T. A new gastric ulcer model induced by ischemia reperfusion in the rat: Role of leukocytes on ulceration in rat stomach. Life Sciences. 1996;**59**(19):295-301

[32] Konturek PC, Brzozowski T, Kania J. Pioglitazone, a specific ligand of peroxisome proliferator-activated receptorgamma, accelerates gastric ulcer healing in rat. European Journal of Pharmacology. 2003;**472**(3):213-220

[33] Naito Y, Yoshikawa T, Yoneta T. A new gastric ulcer model in rats produced by ferrous iron and ascorbic acid injection. Digestion. 1995;**56**(6):472-478

[34] Kaur D, Rana AC, Sharma N, Kumar S. Herbal drugs with antiulcer activity. Journal of Applied Pharmaceutical Science. 2012;**2**(3):160-165

[35] Srinivas TL, Lakshmi SM, Shama SN, Reddy GK, Prasanna KR. Medicinal plants as anti-ulcer agents. Journal of Pharmacognosy and Phytochemistry. 2013;**2**(4):91-97

[36] Schmeda-Hirschmann, G, Yesilada E. Traditional medicine and gastroprotective crude drugs. Journal of Ethnopharmacology. 2005;**100**(1-2):61-66

[37] Vimala G, Shoba GF. A Review on antiulcer activity of few Indian medicinal plants. International Journal of Microbiology. 2014;Article ID 519590, 14 pages

[38] Priyanka A. Some of the medicinal plants with anti-ulcer activity: A review. Journal of Pharmaceutical Science and Research. 2015;**7**(9):772-775

[39] Mehta D. Ulcer-Review on types, anti-ulcer drugs, anti-ulcer medicinal plants, anti-ulcer drug market, diagnostics and current global clinical trials status. Invention and Rapid Pharmacy Practice. 2016;**2**:1-8

[40] Nadkarni's KM. Indian Materia Medica. Popular Prakashan, Mumbai, India. 1976;**1**:9-10

[41] Abd El-Mawla AMA, Osman HEH. Effects of *Gum acacia* aqueous extract on the histology of the intestine and enzymes of both the intestine and the pancreas of albino rats treated with meloxicam. Pharmacognosy Research. 2011;**3**(2):114-121

[42] Maury PK, Jain SK, Lal N, Alok S. A review on antiulcer activity. International Journal of Pharmaceutical Science Research. 2012;**3**(8):2487-2493

[43] Nadkarni's KM. Indian Materia Medica. Popular Prakashan, Mumbai, India. 1976;**1**:38-39

[44] Ilavarasan JR, Monideen S, Vijayalakshmi M. Antiulcer activity of *Aegle marmelos*. Ancient Science of Life. 2002;**21**(4):23-26

[45] Borra SK, Lagisetty RK, Mallela GR. Anti-ulcer effect of *Aloe vera* in non-steroidal anti-inflammatory drug induced peptic ulcers in rats. African Journal of Pharmacy and Pharmacology. 2011;**5**(16):1867-1871

[46] Shaker E, Mahmoud H, Mnaa S. Anti-inflammatory and anti-ulcer activity of the extract from *Alhagi maurorum* (camelthorn). Food and Chemical Toxicology. 2010;**48**:2785-2790

[47] Azamthulla M, Asad M, Prasad VS. Antiulcer activity of *Allium sativum* bulb juice in rats. Saudi Pharmaceutical Journal. 2009;**17**(1):70-77

[48] Mohamed TSS, Pradeep RK, Priyanka N, Madhuri M, Sravanti V, Sarala K. Anti-ulcerogenic effect of aqueous extract of *Annona squamosa* (Linn). International Journal of Research in Phytochemistry and Pharmacology. 2012;**2**(3):157-159

[49] Divakar MC, Rao SB, Nair GRN, Hisham A. The role of fatty acids on the ulcer healing property of the nimbidin fraction of the neem oil. Journal of Medicinal and Aromatic Plants Science. 2001;**23**(3):404-408

[50] Kumar YR, Rajani GP. Analgesic and anti-ulcer activities of ethanol and aqueous extracts of root of *Bauhinia variegate* Linn. International Journal of Pharmacology. 2011;**7**(5):616-622

[51] Nadkarni's KM. Indian Materia Medica. Popular Prakashan, Mumbai, India. 1976; **1**:187-188

[52] Nadkarni's KM. Indian Materia Medica. Popular Prakashan, Mumbai, India. 1976;**1**:197

[53] Indran M, Mahmood AA, Kuppusamy VR. Protective effect of *Carica papaya* L leaf extract against alcohol induced acute gastric damage and blood oxidative stress in rats. West Indian Medical Journal. 2008;**57**(4):323-326

[54] Sairam K, Rao CHV, Goel RK. Effect of *Centella asiatica* Linn on physical and chemical factors induced gastric ulceration and secretion. Indian Journal of Experimental Biology. 2001;**39**:137-142

[55] Inas ZA, Abdallah-Hala AH, Khattab H, Gehan HH. Gastroprotective effect of *Cordia Myxa* L. fruit extract against indomethacin-induced gastric ulceration in rats. Life Sciences Journal. 2011;**8**:433-445

[56] Gregory M, Divya B, Mary RA, Hipolith MMV, Kalaichelvan VK, Palanivel V. Anti-ulcer activity of *Ficus religiosa* leaf ethanolic extract. Asian Pacific Journal of Tropical Biomedicine. 2013;**3**(7):554-556

[57] Khalid MS, Hassan SK, Suresh DK, Hasan R, Saleem MA, Farooqui Z. Antiulcer activity of ethanolic extract of *Gossypium herbaceous* flowers. RGUH. Journal of Pharmaceutical Sciences. 2011;**1**:79S-84S

[58] Srivastava JJ, Gautam H, Sharma S, Rao CV. Anti-ulcer activity of methanol extract of *Hibiscus rosa sinensis* leaves. International Journal of Pharmacy and Pharmaceutical Sciences. 2013;**5**(3):829-830

[59] Ajani EO, Sabiu S, Bamisaye FA, Salami MR, Nurain IO. Ethanolic leaf extract of *Lagenaria brevifolia* (Bitter gourd) inhibits gastric onslaught in indomethacin ulcerated rats. Journal of Applied Biosciences. 2015;**85**:7871-7880

[60] Neelima MS, Patil MB, Lakshmi BVS. Anti-ulcer activity and HPTLC analysis of *Mangifera indica* leaves. International Journal of Pharmaceutical and Phytopharmacological Research. 2012;**1**(4):146-155

[61] Pramod K, Devala RG, Lakshmayya A, Ramachandra SS. GC-MS analysis and antiulcer activity of ethanol extract of tubers of *Momordica tuberosa* Cogn. (cucurbitaceae) in rats. Journal of Applied Pharmacy. 2011;**4**:359-369

[62] Verma VK, Singh N, Saxena P, Singh R. Anti-ulcer and anti-oxidant activity of *Moringa oleifera* (Lam) leaves against aspirin and ethanol induced gastric ulcer in rats. International Research Journal of Pharmacy. 2002;**2**:46-57

[63] Sumbul S, Ahmad MA, Asif M, Saud I, Akhtar M. Evaluation of *Myrtus communis* Linn. berries in experimental ulcer models in rats. Human and Experimental Toxicology. 2010;**29**(11):935-944

[64] Kamble RD, Maske KS, Shaikh HM, Balghare KC, Shikare ON. A review of antiulcer medicinal plants. International Journal of Pharmacy. 2013;**4**(1):78-81

[65] Singh S, Majumdar DK. Evaluation of the gastric antiulcer activity of fixed oil of *Ocimum sanctum* (Holy Basil). Journal of Ethnopharmacology. 1999;**65**(1):13-19

[66] Panchal S, Goswami SS, Shan MB, Santani DD. Effect of *Oryza sativa* bran oil in various experimental ulcer models. Indian Journal of Pharmacology. 2008;**40**(2):146-148

[67] Okoli CO, Ezike AC, Akah PA. Studies on wound healing and antiulcer activities of extract of aerial parts of *Phyllanthus niruri* L. (Euphorbiaceae). American Journal of Pharmacology and Toxicology. 2009;**4**(4):118-126

[68] Umana EU, Timbuak JA, Musa SA, Ikyembe DT, Abdurrashid S, Hamman WO. Ulceroprotective effect of methanol extract of *Psidium guajava* leaves on ethanol induced gastric ulcer in adult wistar rats. Asian Journal of Medical Sciences. 2012;**4**(2):75-78

[69] Ahmad H, Wadud A, Jahan N, Khazir M, Sofi G. Evaluation of anti-ulcer activity of hydro alcoholic extract of Post Sumaq (*Rhus coriaria* Linn.) in ethanol induced gastric ulcer in experimental rats. International Research Journal of Medical Sciences. 2013;**1**(10):7-12

[70] Bhalke RD, Giri MA, Anarthe SJ, Pal SC. Antiulcer activity of the ethanol extract of leaves of *Sesbania grandiflora* (Linn.). International Journal of Pharmacy and Pharmaceutical Sciences. 2010;**2**(4):206-208

[71] Khan I, Nisar M, Ebad F, Nadeem S, Saeed M, Khan H. Anti-inflammatory activities of sieboldogenin from *Smilax china* Linn.: Experimental and com putational studies. Journal of Ethnopharmacology. 2009;**121**:175-177

[72] Kavitha GGS, Parvathi S, Ramkumar PSS, Shanmuga SP. Pharmacological and phytochemical evaluation of anti-ulcerogenic potential of *Solanum nigrum.* Indian Journal of Pharmaceutical Science and Research. 2012;**3**(8):2837-2840

[73] Saheed S, Taofeeq G, Taofik OS, Emmanuel OA, Abdulhakeem S, Ismaila NI, Abdulazeez B. Indomethacin-induced gastric ulceration in rats: Protective roles of *Spondias mombin* and *Ficus exasperate*. Toxicology Report. 2015;**2**:261-267

[74] Kumar S, Suman S, Sharma S, Kalra P. Antiulcer effect of the methanolic extract of *Tamarindus indica* seeds in different experimental models. Journal of Pharmacy and Bioallied Sciences. 2011;**2**(3):236-241

[75] Raju D, Ilango K, Chitra V, Ashish K. Evaluation of antiulcer activity of methanolic extract of *Terminalia chebula* fruits in experimental rats. Journal of Pharmaceutical Sciences and Research. 2009;**1**(3):101-107

[76] Bandyopadhyay U,Biswas K, Sengupta A, Moitra P, Dutta P, Sarkar D, Debnath P, Ganguly CK, Banerjee RK. Clinical studies on the effect of Neem (*Azadirachta indica*) bark extract on gastric secretion and gastroduodenal ulcer. Life Sciences. 2004;**75**(24):2867-2878

[77] Michael BA, Charles A, Isaac G, Alexander N. *In vivo* models used for evaluation of potential antigastroduodenal ulcer agents. *Ulcers*, 2013. Article ID 796405, 12 pages

[78] Kadiri M, Ojewumi AW, Kokumo YO. Ethnobotanical study of plants used in managing ulcer in Abeokuta metropolis, Ogun State, Nigeria. Journal of Natural Science, Engineering and Technology. 2013;**12**:76-88

[79] Alebiosu CO, Ugwah OM, Ugwah-Oguejiofor CJ, Njan AA. Ethno botanical studies of medicinal plants used in the management of Peptic ulcer disease in Sokoto State, North Western Nigeria. International Research Journal of Pharmacy and Pharmacology. 2012;**2**(9):225-230

[80] Sabiu S, O'neill FH, Ashafa AOT. *Zea mays, Stigma maydis* prevents and extenuates acetaminophen-perturbed oxidative onslaughts in rat hepatocytes. Pharmaceutical Biology, 2016;**54**(11): 2664-2673. DOI: http://dx.doI.org/10.1080/13880209.20161178307

[81] Ajani EO, Sabiu S, Bamisaye FA, Adenigba BV, Awomoyi DD, Adeyanju MM. Hepatoprotective and antioxidative effect of ethanolic leaf extract of *Langenaria breviflora* (bitter gourd) on indomethacin-ulcerated rats. IOSR Journal of Pharmacy and Biological Science. 2014;**9**(5 V I):61-68

[82] Hong Y, Xingchang P, Zhixiu S, Shaokang W, Ligang Y, Guiju S. Protective effect of wheat peptides against indomethacin-induced oxidative stress in IEC-6 cells. Nutrients. 2014;**6**:564-574

[83] Dae YC, Jin IK, Soo-Heon P, Jae KK. Proanthocyanidin from grape seed extracts protects indomethacin-induced small intestinal mucosal injury. Gastroenterology Research Practice. 2014;**14**:618-626

[84] Bjornsson E. Review article: Drug-induced liver injury in clinical practice. Alimentary Pharmacology Therapeutics. 2013;**32**:3-13

[85] Jarupongprapa S, Ussavasodhi P, Katchamart W. Comparison of gastrointestinal adverse effects between cyclooxygenase-2 inhibitors and non-selective, non-steroidal anti-inflammatory drugs plus proton pump inhibitors: A systematic review and meta-analysis. Journal of Gastroenterology. 2013;**48**:830-838

[86] Kang HS, Ock J, Lee HJ, Lee YJ, Kwon BM, Hong SH. Early growth response protein-1-upregulation and nuclear translocation by 2′-benzoyloxycinnamaldehyde induces prostate cancer cell death. Cancer Letter. 2013;**329**:217-227

[87] Vaish V, Piplani H, Rana C, Vaiphei K, Sanyal SN. NSAIDs may regulate EGR-1- mediated induction of reactive oxygen species and non-steroidal anti-inflammatory drug-induced gene (NAG)-1 to initiate intrinsic pathway of apoptosis for the chemoprevention of colorectal cancer. Molecular Cell Biochemistry. 2013;**378**:47-64

[88] Valko M, Leibfritz D, Moncol J, Cronin MTD, Mazur M, Telser J. Free radicals and antioxidants in normal physiological functions and human disease. International Journal of Biochemistray and Cell Biology. 2007;**39**:44-84

[89] Sabiu S, Wudil AM. Comparative effects of *Telfaira occidentalis* and *Vernonia amygdalina* on garlic-induced hepatotoxicity in rats. Biological and Environmental Sciences Journal for the Tropics. 2011;**8**(4):193-197

[90] Shu YZ. Recent natural products based drug development: A pharmaceutical industry perspective. Journal of Natural Product. 1998;**61**:1053-1107

Chapter 4

Gastric Antral Vascular Ectasia and Portal Hypertensive Gastropathy

Daryl Ramai, Sandar Linn and Madhavi Reddy

Additional information is available at the end of the chapter

http://dx.doi.org/10.5772/intechopen.70610

Abstract

Gastric antral vascular ectasia (GAVE) and portal hypertensive gastropathy (PHG) are mucosal lesions that can cause chronic gastrointestinal bleeding in the patients with cirrhosis. While PHG occurs exclusively in patients with liver cirrhosis, GAVE can also present in patients with systemic and autoimmune conditions. The need to accurately characterize these two conditions is dependent on clinical, endoscopic, and histological parameters. The management of GAVE utilizes endoscopic ablation techniques, while medical therapy is directed toward stabilizing portal pressure in patients with PHG. Herein, we review the epidemiology, diagnosis, pathophysiology, and medical, endoscopic, and surgical management of GAVE and PHG.

Keywords: stomach diseases, gastric antral vascular ectasia (GAVE), portal hypertensive gastropathy (PHG), portal hypertension, cirrhosis, management

1. Introduction

Gastric antral vascular ectasia (GAVE) and portal hypertensive gastropathy (PHG) are common gastric mucosal lesions that occur in patients with portal hypertension. These two conditions are responsible for acute on chronic gastrointestinal bleeding. While these two clinical entities share similar clinical presentations, their underlying pathophysiology, endoscopic features, and management options are different. The pathophysiology of GAVE is related to local changes in gastric mucosa, and management is aimed at endoscopic reduction of blood loss using thermal therapies. The pathophysiology of PHG is related to portal hypertension, and management is aimed at reducing portal hypertension using pharmacologic and in some cases portosystemic shunts. Thus, it is important to differentiate GAVE and PHG as their management options are different.

2. Epidemiology

GAVE accounts for approximately 4% of all upper gastrointestinal bleeding [1]. Approximately 40% of GAVE patients have cirrhosis of the liver, and 1 in 40 patients require liver transplantation [2]. Cirrhotic GAVE patients are predominantly males (75%; mean age 65 years), whereas noncirrhotic GAVE patients are predominantly females (71%; mean age of 73 years). GAVE has been associated with autoimmune disorders such as autoimmune connective tissue disorders (62%), Raynaud's phenomenon (31%), and sclerodactyly (20%) [3]. GAVE have also been reported in other medical conditions including scleroderma, bone marrow transplantation, chronic renal failure, ischemic heart disease, hypertension, valvular heart disease, familial Mediterranean fever, and acute myeloid leukemia [3–6].

The prevalence of PHG varies from 20 to 75% in portal hypertensive patients, and from 35 to 80% in patients with cirrhosis [7]. According to the HALT-C trial, approximately 37% of patients (364 of 1011) with biopsy confirmed cirrhosis or bridging fibrosis from hepatitis C had PHG [8]. While PHG can present at any age, its severity can vary from mild to severe. The severity of liver disease and severity of portal hypertension greatly influences the natural progression of PHG [9].

3. Pathophysiology

The pathophysiology of GAVE remains unknown; however, several mechanisms have been proposed including gastric dysmotility or autoimmune reactivity to gastric blood vessels [10–12]. A study on antral motility revealed an increase in antral area transit time with cirrhosis and GAVE when compared to controls [10]. Chronic recurrent trauma can lead to fibromuscular hyperplasia and vascular ectasia. Reduced gastrin levels have also been identified in GAVE patients when compared to patients with severe PTH and normal controls [13]. Prostaglandins E2 (PGE2) levels were found significantly elevated when compared to controls [14]. GAVE is not associated with portal hypertension and treatments aimed to decrease portal pressure have no role in treatment of GAVE [15].

The pathogenesis of PHG is related to increased resistance to portal blood flow in patients with liver disease, and concomitant elevation in portal pressure [16]. In patients with portal hypertension, approximately 70% develop PHG [17]. Resolution of PHG and its recurrence has been observed in patients with cirrhosis posttransjugular intrahepatic portosystemic shunt (TIPS) placement, and in noncirrhotic patients with postsurgical decompression of the portal system [17–19]. However, the linear correlation between the severity of portal hypertension and that of PHG is controversial. In a prospective study of 331 patients, it was reported that severe PHG showed a significantly shorter expected survival time than mild PHG (median survival time, 77.6 ± 9.6 months in severe PHG) [20]. The study concluded that PHG was associated with severity of portal hypertension and prognosis in patients with cirrhosis. However, other studies have been unable to demonstrate a correlation between the severity of portal hypertension and that of PHG [21–23].

Other molecular mediators at the mucosal level have been implicated in the development of PHG including tumor necrosis factor (TNF)-α, endothelin-1 (ET-1), nitric oxide (NO), and prostaglandins [21, 24]. Interestingly, patients with cirrhosis and PHG have abnormal blood circulation, which makes them susceptible to reduced delivery of oxygen to the gastric mucosa [21, 25]. This phenomenon modifies blood circulation which enables reduced resistance of gastric mucosa to irritants in patients with cirrhosis and portal hypertension [26].

4. Diagnostic evaluation

GAVE and PHG can be encountered during upper endoscopy in both symptomatic and asymptomatic patients with liver cirrhosis. GI bleeding is the common significant complication of GAVE and PHG. PHG is responsible for about 8% of nonvariceal upper GI bleeding, while GAVE accounts for up to 4% [27, 28]. Both GAVE and PHG may have similar endoscopic appearances and require further histological analysis. In 1995, Payne et al. established that portal hypertensive gastropathy (PHG) and GAVE are distinct clinical entities that require different forms of treatments [13]. Thus, it is incumbent on clinicians to be able to differentiate both diseases.

GAVE is a disease limited to the stomach and is almost exclusively noted in the gastric antrum on endoscopy [29]. GAVE was first reported in 1984 and initially termed 'watermelon' stomach in three patients with iron deficiency anemia [30]. In their report, they described visible convoluted and tortuous columns of ectatic vessels along rugal folds of the antrum, which converged at the pylorus, resembling stripes of a watermelon. In more severe cases, GAVE can present as more punctate lesions or more diffusely, extending to the gastric body, which is most commonly associated with GAVE in cirrhotics than other etiologies [31]. Interestingly, GAVE patients have been reported to have more severe liver disease, greater blood loss, lower serum gastrin levels, and a higher incidence of previous sclerotherapy [13].

Histologically, GAVE is characterized by dilated mucosal capillaries and venules with intimal thickening, fibrin thrombi, spindle cell proliferation, and fibromuscular hyperplasia of the lamina propria [13, 32]. The presence of these histological features is used to calculate a GAVE score which has 80% diagnostic accuracy. This can be used to distinguish GAVE from PHG with a GAVE score equal or greater than three [13].

PHG lesions are typically seen in the gastric fundus unlike GAVE which is commonly found in the antrum. Endoscopically, PHG appears as a mosaic-like pattern or a diffuse, erythematous, and reticular cobblestone pattern of gastric mucosa consisting of small polygonal areas with superimposed red punctate lesions >2 mm in diameter and a depressed white border [33–35]. Severe PHG is associated with flat or bulging red spots, resembling a scarlatina rash with friability or diffuse hemorrhagic gastropathy [36–38].

5. Management of GAVE

5.1. Endoscopic management

The treatment of choice in managing patients with GAVE is endoscopic ablation of the lesions. Pharmacologic or surgical intervention should be considered when endoscopic therapy has failed. Argon plasma coagulation (APC) has become the method most utilized by endoscopist. APC is a noncontact technique that uses argon gas to equally distribute thermal energy. High-frequency current is applied to the tissue with controllable depth of coagulation (roughly 2–3 mm) [39]. Its efficacy ranges from 90 to 100% [40]. Endoscopic band ligation (EBL) and radiofrequency ablation (RFA) are newer and promising techniques in the treatment of GAVE; however, RFA requires additional training and is not readily available in all endoscopic centers [41].

Compared to older laser therapy methods, APC is more user-friendly, manageable, cheaper, and safer. The risk of perforation is very low and limited to very thin-walled structures [42]. The pooled recurrence rate of bleeding is estimated at 36% [43]. Cryotherapy has also been introduced as another means for managing GAVE. It makes use of nitrous oxide to freeze abnormal mucosa and causes superficial necrosis. A pilot study that assessed 12 patients with GAVE and anemia showed that 50% of patients achieved a complete response after cryotherapy [44]. The remaining patients achieved a partial response with decreased transfusion requirements. However, the optimal delivery mechanism and the number of treatments required remain unclear.

Overall, EBL seems to be the safest and has only been associated with minor complications such as abdominal pain [45]. An observational study of 22 patients (9 patients receiving endoscopic thermal therapy vs. 9 patients receiving EBL) reported fewer bleeding in the EBL cohort (67 vs. 23%), as well as fewer treatment sessions for EBL (4.9 vs. 1.9), and a decrease in EBL-related transfusions (−5.2 vs. −12.7) [46]. A prospective study of 21 patients reported a clinical response that was achieved in 19 patients (91%) after a mean of 2.28 endoscopic sessions and a mean of 16 bands applied [47]. Another study comparing the efficacy of EBL vs. APC reported a lower recurrence rate in the EBL cohort (8.3 vs. 68%) [48].

5.2. Medical treatment

While a variety of drugs have been used to manage GAVE-related bleeding, none has shown to be clinically effective and efficacious as an alternative to invasive methods. Pilot studies with estrogen-progesterone hormone therapy have been shown to control bleeding due to gastrointestinal vascular malformations, including GAVE, with side effects [49–51]. Despite bleeding cessation, GAVE lesions persisted. Reduction of treatment frequency resulted in bleeding relapse, requiring reinstitution of daily therapy for hemostatic control [49, 52, 53]. However, this form of treatment is not well studied and patients are at risk for developing severe side effects, such as menorrhagia and gynecomastia, and increased risk of endometrial and breast cancer [54].

A long acting somatostatin analog, octreotide, has been reported as an effective drug in controlling chronic bleeding due to vascular abnormalities [55]. This may in part be due to the inhibitory effect on neuroendocrine cells, ectatic vessels, and smooth muscle cells [55, 56]. Octreotide also displays antiangiogenic effects and limits the growth of blood vessels [57]. However, octreotide treatment has been unsuccessfully replicated by other authors and thus necessitates further investigation [58]. Success has been reported from the use of corticosteroids, tranexamic acid, thalidomide, and serotonin antagonist [59–63]. However, these treatments have been reported in some case reports and the results have not been confirmed by controlled clinical trials.

5.3. Surgical intervention

Surgical intervention is reserved for patients who do not respond to medical and endoscopic therapies. Surgical approaches include gastrectomy and antrectomy, which may be the only reliable approach to achieving a cure. Antrectomy is more commonly used and has clinical efficacy in eliminating bleeding and transfusion dependency, as patients do not report postoperative recurrence of bleeding was associated with multiorgan failure [64]. Portacaval shunts and TIPS have no role in the management of GAVE [11]. In GAVE patients due to underlying cirrhosis, complete resolution of symptoms has been observed following liver transplant, despite persistent portal hypertension [15].

6. Management of PHG

6.1. Medical treatment

The management of PHG is focused on abating portal pressure, mainly through the use of medical therapy rather than endoscopic means. Similar to esophageal varices, management attempts to reduce hepatic venous pressure gradient (HVPG) to <12 mmHg or by 20% which correlates with a reduction in mortality in some studies [65]. A meta-analysis established that target HVPG is a valid marker to monitor drug efficacy for variceal bleeding and patient prognosis [65]. Beta blockers are first-line drugs used to reduce portal pressure and have the most benefit in patients with mild PHG [66]. Modest effects have been noted in patients with severe PHG [67]. It is unclear whether beta blockers are prophylactically effective in preventing bleeding from PHG [24]. However, in patients receiving propranolol or nadolol for esophageal variceal bleeding prophylaxis, beta blocker therapy showed a reduction in future PHG bleeding [68].

In a randomized controlled trial to investigate the efficacy of propranolol, 26 of 54 patients received propranolol and the rest placebo. Daily doses of 40–320 mg were used. In the cohort receiving propranolol, patients reported significantly lower rates of rebleeding (38 vs. 65%) at 12 months and at 30 months (7 vs. 52%) compared with controls [67]. Similarly, a smaller study using a dose of 24–480 mg/day decreased the incidence of acute bleeding in 16 patients with PHG and also reduced the grade of PHG in 24 asymptomatic patients when given at a dose of 160 mg/day [68].

In unstable patients who have contraindications for beta blockers, other agents have been studied with varying efficacy including somatostatin, octreotide, terlipressin, and vasopressin [69–72]. Somatostatin and its analogs showed complete control of acute bleeding with 11% rebleeding after withdrawing infusion [69]. Octreotide controlled bleeding in 100% of patients within 48 h. Vasopressin controlled bleeding in 64% of patients over the same time [71]. Terlipressin, a vasopressin analog (not available in the United States), was similarly effective as vasopressin [72].

6.2. Endoscopic management

Acute bleeding in the setting of PHG rarely occurs. A large study reported an incidence of acute bleeding from gastropathy in 8 of 315 patients (2.5%), compared to chronic bleeding which occurred in 34 patients (10.8%) [73]; however, if it occurs, such bleeding episodes can be severe and challenging to manage. In addition to intravenous medical therapy with aforementioned agents aimed at reducing portal pressure and hemostatic control, appropriate antibiotic and resuscitation should be initiated and tailored to the patient's needs.

Endoscopic therapy for acute bleeding from PHG remains investigational and may provide temporary control. For patients with refractory bleeding who are not candidates for portosystemic shunting, limited data suggest that endoscopic thermal therapy may be efficacious. Similar to GAVE, APC has proven successful in controlling bleeding and reducing transfusion requirements [74]. Furthermore, hemostatic powder is emerging as a useful means for managing patients with acute bleeding. The powder acts by forming a barrier over the bleeding site and increasing the concentration of clotting factors [75].

6.3. Surgical intervention

In cases of failed medical or endoscopic therapy requiring increase blood transfusions, portosystemic shunt therapy should be considered through the placement of a transjugular intrahepatic portosystemic shunt (TIPS). Shunting works by relieving portal hypertension with the placement of a tube (shunt) between the portal vein which carries blood from the intestines to the liver and the hepatic vein which carries blood from the liver back to the heart. Patients who have the TIPS procedure show significant improvement in endoscopic appearance of PHG and number of transfusion requirements [76].

A prospective study of 30 patients with mild PHG and 10 patients with severe PHG with recurrent GI bleeding had a 75% reduction in endoscopic severity, a Childs-Pugh Score of 11.5, and a mean reduction in portacaval gradient from 20 to 12 mmHg following TIPS [17]. Patients typically show endoscopic improvement in 6 weeks for mild cases and up to 3 months for more severe cases of PHG [77]. A retrospective study of 40 Child-Pugh class A and B cirrhotic patients comparing surgical shunting and TIPS found improved outcomes from surgical shunting with reduced 30-day mortality, reduced rebleeding events, and fewer shunt revisions and hospitalizations [78].

However, surgical shunting carries risks of substantial perioperative morbidity and mortality. In those who survive operation, accelerated hepatic decompensation and neuropsychologic deterioration (portosystemic encephalopathy) significantly diminish the overall benefit of the shunting procedure [78]. Similarly, TIPS carries a potential risk for rapid liver failure necessitating liver transplantation [79].

7. Conclusion

In summary, GAVE and PHG are two clinically distinct entities that present with gastrointestinal blood loss. Majority of patients with portal hypertension and cirrhosis will develop PHG; however, it can also occur in the setting of noncirrhotic portal hypertension. GAVE is associated with gastric dysmotility, autoimmune reactivity, reduced gastrin levels, and elevated prostaglandins. It is not associated with cirrhosis. Therapy of PHG is directed toward lowering and stabilizing portal pressure with beta blockers or shunt procedures. GAVE management mainly involves the use of endoscopic methods to ablate bleeding lesions. When GAVE is complicated by cirrhosis, it is incumbent on clinicians to differentiate it from PHG as GAVE does not respond to treatments aimed at reduction of portal pressure.

Author details

Daryl Ramai[1,2]*, Sandar Linn[1] and Madhavi Reddy[1]

*Address all correspondence to: dramai@sgu.edu

1 Department of Gastroenterology and Hepatology, The Brooklyn Hospital Center – Clinical Affiliate of The Mount Sinai Hospital, Brooklyn, New York, USA

2 Department of Anatomical Sciences, St George's University School of Medicine, True Blue, Grenada, West Indies

References

[1] Dulai GS, Jensen DM, Kovacs TO, et al. Endoscopic treatment outcomes in watermelon stomach patients with and without portal hypertension. Endoscopy. 2004;**36**:68-72

[2] Ward EM, Raimondo M, Rosser BG, et al. Prevalence and natural history of gastric antral vascular ectasia (GAVE) in patients undergoing orthoptic liver transplantation. Journal of Clinical Gastroenterology. 2004;**38**:898-900

[3] Gostout CJ, Viggiano TR, Ahlquist DA, et al. The clinical and endoscopic spectrum of the watermelon stomach. Journal of Clinical Gastroenterology. 1992;**15**:256-263

[4] Tobin RW, Hackman RC, Kimmey MB, et al. Bleeding from gastric antral vascular ectasia in marrow transplant patients. Gastrointestinal Endoscopy. 1996;**44**:223-229

[5] Sebastian S, O'Morain CA, Buckley MJ. Review article: Current therapeutic options for gastric antral vascular ectasia. Alimentary Pharmacology & Therapeutics. 2003;**18**:157-165

[6] Takahashi T, Takuya M, Oki M, et al. Severe hemorrhage from gastric antral vascular ectasia developed in a patient with AML. International Journal of Hematology. 2006;**83**:467-468

[7] Gjeorgjievski M, Cappell MS. Portal hypertensive gastropathy: A systematic review of the pathophysiology, clinical presentation, natural history and therapy. World Journal of Hepatology. 2016;**8**:231-262

[8] Fontana RJ, Sanyal AJ, Ghany MG, et al. Development and progression of portal hypertensive gastropathy in patients with chronic hepatitis C. The American Journal of Gastroenterology. 2011;**106**:884-893

[9] Merli M, Nicolini G, Angeloni S, et al. The natural history of portal hypertensive gastropathy in patients with liver cirrhosis and mild portal hypertension. The American Journal of Gastroenterology. 2004;**99**:1959-1965

[10] Charneau J, Petit R, Cales P, et al. Antral motility in patients with cirrhosis with or without gastric antral vascular ectasia. Gut. 1995;**37**:488-492

[11] Spahr L, Villeneuve JP, Dufresne MP, et al. Gastric antral vascular ectasia in cirrhotic patients: Absence of relation with portal hypertension. Gut. 1999;**44**:739-742

[12] Watson M, Hally RJ, McCue PA, Varga J, Jimenez SA. Gastric antral vascular ectasia (watermelon stomach) in patients with systemic sclerosis. Arthritis & Rheumatology. 1996;**39**:341-346

[13] Payen JL, Cales P, Voigt JJ, et al. Severe portal hypertensive gastropathy and antral vascular ectasia are distinct entities in patients with cirrhosis. Gastroenterology. 1995; **108**:138-144

[14] Saperas E, Perez Ayuso RM, Poca E, et al. Increased gastric PGE2 biosynthesis in cirrhotic patients with gastric vascular ectasia. The American Journal of Gastroenterology. 1990;**85**:138-144

[15] Vincent C, Pomier-Layrargues G, Dagenais M, et al. Cure of gastric antral vascular ectasia by liver transplantation despite persistent portal hypertension: A clue for pathogenesis. Liver Transplantation. 2002;**8**:717-720

[16] Ferraz JG, Wallace JL. Underlying mechanisms of portal hypertensive gastropathy. Journal of Clinical Gastroenterology. 1997;**25**(Suppl 1):S73-S78

[17] Kamath PS, Lacerda M, Ahlquist DA, et al. Gastric mucosal responses to intrahepatic portosystemic shunting in patients with cirrhosis. Gastroenterology. 2000;**118**:905-911

[18] de Melo MR, de Figueiredo JL, AraújoFilho JL, et al. Portal hypertension in mansonic schistosomiasis: Repercussions of surgical treatment on the histomorphometric profile of the gastric mucosa. Revista daSociedadeBrasileirade Medicina Tropical. 2007;**40**:71-75

[19] Soin AS, Acharya SK, Mathur M, et al. Portal hypertensive gastropathy in non-cirrhotic patients. The effect of lienorenal shunts. Journal of Clinical Gastroenterology. 1998;**26**:64-67

[20] Kim MY, Choi H, Baik SK, et al. Portal hypertensive gastropathy: Correlation with portal hypertension and prognosis in cirrhosis. Digestive Diseases and Science. 2010; **55**:3561-3567

[21] Ohta M, Hashizume M, Higashi H, et al. Portal and gastric mucosal hemodynamics in cirrhotic patients with portal-hypertensive gastropathy. Hepatology. 1994;**20**:1432-1436

[22] Sarin SK, Lahoti D, Saxena SP, et al. Prevalence, classification and natural history of gastric varices: A long-term follow-up study in 568 portal hypertension patients. Hepatology. 1992;**16**:1343-1349

[23] Panes J, Bordas JM, Pique JM, et al. Increased gastric mucosal perfusion in cirrhotic patients with portal hypertensive gastropathy. Gastroenterology. 1992;**103**:1875-1882

[24] Cubillas R, Rockey DC. Portal hypertensive gastropathy: A review. Liver International. 2010;**30**:1094-1102

[25] Curvelo LA, Brabosa W, Rhor R, et al. Underlying mechanism of portal hypertensive gastropathy in cirrhosis: A hemodynamic and morphological approach. Journal of Gastroenterology and Hepatology. 2009;**24**:1541-1546

[26] Sarfeh IJ, Soliman H, Waxman K, et al. Impaired oxygenation of gastric mucosa in portal hypertension. The basis for increased susceptibility to injury. Digestive Diseases and Science. 1989;**34**:225-228

[27] Gostout CJ, Viggiano TR, Balm RK. Acute gastrointestinal bleeding from portal hypertensive gastropathy: Prevalence and clinical features. American Journal of Gastroenterology. 1993;**88**:2030-2033

[28] Dulai GS, Jensen DM, Kovacs TO, et al. Endoscopic treatment outcomes in watermelon stomach patients with and without portal hypertension. Endoscopy. 2004;**36**:68-72

[29] Burak KW, Beck PL. Portal hypertensive gastropathy and gastric antral vascular ectasia (GAVE) syndrome. Gut. 2001;**49**:866-872

[30] Jabbari M, Cherry R, Lough JO, et al. Gastric antral vascular ectasia: The watermelon stomach. Gastroenterology. 1984;**87**:1165-1170

[31] Ito M, Uchida Y, Kamano S, et al. Clinical comparisons between two subsets of gastric antral vascular ectasia. Gastrointestinal Endoscopy. 2001;**53**:764-770

[32] Suit PF, Petras RE, Bauer TW, Petrini JL. Gastric antral vascular ectasia. A histologic and morphometric study of the watermelon stomach. The American Journal of Surgical Pathology. 1987;**11**:750-757

[33] Kamath PS, Shah VH. Portal hypertension and bleeding esophageal varices. In: Boyer TD, Manns MP, Sanyal AJ, editors. Zakim and Boyer's Hepatology: A Textbook of Liver Disease. 6th ed. Philadelphia: Elsevier Saunders; 2012. p. 296-326

[34] Feldman M, Lee EL. Gastritis. In: Feldman M, Friedman LS, Brandt LJ, editors. Sleisenger and Fordtran's Gastrointestinal and Liver Disease: Pathophysiology, Diagnosis, Management. 10th ed. Philadelphia: Elsevier Saunders; 2010. p. 868-883

[35] Vigneri S, Termini R, Piraino A, et al. The stomach in liver cirrhosis. Endoscopic, morphological, and clinical correlations. Gastroenterology. 1991;**101**:472-478

[36] Thuluvath PJ, Yoo HY. Portal hypertensive gastropathy. American Journal of Gastroenterology. 2002;**97**:2973-2978

[37] Thuluvath PJ. Management of upper gastrointestinal hemorrhage related to portal hypertension. In: Yamada T, Alpers DH, Kalloo AN, Kaplowitz N, Owyang C, Powell DW, editors. Textbook of Gastroenterology. 5th ed. Oxford, UK: Wiley-Blackwell; 2009. p. 2897-3017

[38] Bhattacharya B. Non-neoplastic disorders of the stomach. In: Iacobuzio-Donahue CA, Montgomery E, Goldblum JR, editors. Gastrointestinal and Liver Pathology. 2nd ed. Philadelphia: Elsevier Saunders; 2012. p. 65-141

[39] Yusoff I, Brennan F, Ormonde D, Laurence B. Argon plasma coagulation for the treatment of watermelon stomach. Endoscopy. 2002;**34**:407-410

[40] Roman S, Saurin JC, Dumortier J, et al. Tolerance and efficacy of argon plasma coagulation for controlling bleeding in patients with typical and atypical manifestations of watermelon stomach. Endoscopy. 2003;**35**:1024-1028

[41] Dray X, Repici A, Gonzalez P, et al. Radiofrequency ablation for the treatment of gastric antral vascular ectasia. Endoscopy. 2014;**46**:963-969

[42] Wahab PJ, Mulder CJ, den Hartog G, Thies JE. Argon plasma coagulation in flexible gastrointestinal endoscopy: Pilot experiences. Endoscopy 1997;**29**:176-181

[43] Jackson CS, Gerson LB. Management of gastrointestinal angiodysplastic lesions (GIADs): A systematic review and meta-analysis. American Journal of Gastroenterology. 2014;**109**:474-483

[44] Cho S, Zanati S, Yong E, et al. Endoscopic cryotherapy for the management of gastric antral vascular ectasia. Gastrointestinal Endoscopy. 2008;**68**:895-902

[45] Zepeda-Gomez S. Endoscopic treatment for gastric antral vascular ectasia: Current options. GE-Portuguese Journal of Gastroenterology. 2017;**24**:176-182

[46] Wells CD, Harrison ME, Gurudu SR, et al. Treatment of gastric antral vascular ectasia (watermelon stomach) with endoscopic band ligation. Gastrointestinal Endoscopy. 2008;**68**:231-236

[47] Zepeda-Gomez S, Sultanian R, Teshima C, et al. Gastric antral vascular ectasia: A prospective study of treatment with endoscopic band ligation. Endoscopy. 2015;**47**:538-540

[48] Sato T, Yamazaki K, Akaike J. Endoscopic band ligation versus argon plasma coagulation for gastric antral vascular ectasia associated with liver diseases. Digestive Endoscopy. 2012;**24**:237-242

[49] Manning RJ. Estrogen/progesterone treatment of diffuse antral vascular ectasia. American Journal of Gastroenterology. 1995;**90**:154-156

[50] Tran A, Villeneuve JP, Bilodeau M, et al. Treatment of chronic bleeding from gastric antral vascular ectasia (GAVE) with estrogen-progesterone in cirrhotic patients: An open pilot study. American Journal of Gastroenterology. 1999;**94**:2909-2911

[51] van Cutsem E, Rutgeerts P, Vantrappen G. Treatment of bleeding gastrointestinal vascular malformations with oestrogen-progesterone. Lancet 1990;**335**:953-955

[52] Schoonbroodt D, Horsmans Y, Hoang P, et al. Vascular gastric anomalies, CREST syndrome and primary biliary cirrhosis: Efficacy of ethinyl estradiol-norethisterone combination. Gastroenterologie Clinique etBiologique. 1994;**18**:649-651

[53] Moss SF, Ghosh P, Thomas DM, Jackson JE, Calam J. Gastric antral vascular ectasia: Maintenance treatment with oestrogen-progesterone. Gut. 1992;**33**:715-717

[54] Grady D, Rubin SM, Petitti DB, et al. Hormone therapy to prevent disease and prolong life in postmenopausal women. Annals of Internal Medicine. 1992;**117**:1016-1037

[55] Nardone G, Rocco A, Balzano T. The efficacy of octreotide therapy in chronic bleeding due to vascular abnormalities of the gastrointestinal tract. Alimentary Pharmacology & Therapeutics. 1999;**13**:1429-1363

[56] Li SC, Martijn C, Cui T, et al. The somatostatin analogue octreotide inhibits growth of small intestine neuroendocrine tumour cells. PloS One. 2012;**7**:e48411

[57] Zalatnai A, Timar F. Vitro antiangiogenic effect of sandostatin (octreotide) on the proliferation of the placental vessels. Anticancer Research. 2002;**22**:4225-4227

[58] Barbara G, De Giorgio R, Salvioli B, et al. Unsuccessful octreotide treatment of the watermelon stomach. Journal of Clinical Gastroenterology. 1998;**26**:345-346

[59] Bhowmick BK. Watermelon stomach treated with oral corticosteroid. Journal of the Royal Society of Medicine. 1993;**86**:52

[60] Suzuki T, Hirano M, Oka H. Long-term corticosteroid therapy for gastric antral vascular ectasia. American Journal of Gastroenterology. 1996;**91**:1873-1874

[61] McCormick PA, Ooi H, Crosbie O. Tranexamic acid for severe bleeding gastric antral vascular ectasia in cirrhosis. Gut. 1998;**42**:750-752

[62] Dunne KA, Hill J, Dillon JF. Treatment of chronic transfusion-dependent gastric antral vascular ectasia (watermelon stomach) with thalidomide. European Journal of Gastroenterology & Hepatology. 2006;**18**:455-456

[63] Cabral JE, Pontes JM, Toste M, et al. Watermelon stomach: Treatment with a serotonin antagonist. American Journal of Gastroenterology. 1991;**86**:927-928

[64] Novitsky YW, Kercher KW, Czerniach DR, Litwin DE. Watermelon stomach: Pathophysiology, diagnosis, and management. Journal of Gastrointestinal Surgery. 2003;**7**: 652-661

[65] Albillos A, Banares R, Gonzalez M, et al. Value of the hepatic venous pressure gradient to monitor drug therapy for portal hypertension: A meta-analysis. American Journal of Gastroenterology. 2007;**102**:1116-1126

[66] Hosking SW, Kennedy HJ, Seddon I, Triger DR. The role of propranolol in congestive gastropathy of portal hypertension. Hepatology. 1987;**7**:437-441

[67] Perez-Ayuso RM, Pique JM, Bosch J, et al. Propranolol in prevention of recurrent bleeding from severe portal hypertensive gastropathy in cirrhosis. Lancet. 1991;**337**:1431-1434

[68] Lo GH, Lai KH, Cheng JS, et al. The effects of endoscopic variceal ligation and propranolol on portal hypertensive gastropathy: A prospective, controlled trial. Gastrointestinal Endoscopy. 2001;**53**:579-584

[69] Kouroumalis EA, Koutroubakis IE, Manousos ON. Somatostatin for acute severe bleeding from portal hypertensive gastropathy. European Journal of Gastroenterology & Hepatology. 1998;**10**:509-512

[70] Panes J, Pique JM, Bordas JM, et al. Effect of bolus injection and continuous infusion of somatostatin on gastric perfusion in cirrhotic patients with portal-hypertensive gastropathy. Hepatology. 1994;**20**:336-341

[71] Zhou Y, Qiao L, Wu J, et al. Comparison of the efficacy of octreotide, vasopressin, and omeprazole in the control of acute bleeding in patients with portal hypertensive gastropathy: A controlled study. Journal of Gastroenterology & Hepatology. 2002;**17**:973-979

[72] Bruha R, Marecek Z, Spicak J, et al. Double-blind randomized, comparative multicenter study of the effect of terlipressin in the treatment of acute esophageal variceal and/or hypertensive gastropathy bleeding. Hepato-Gastroenterology. 2002;**49**:1161-1166

[73] Primignani M, Carpinelli L, Preatoni P, et al. Natural history of portal hypertensive gastropathy in patients with liver cirrhosis. The new Italian endoscopic Club for the study and treatment of esophageal varices (NIEC). Gastroenterology. 2000;**119**:181-187

[74] Herrera S, Bordas JM, Llach J, et al. The beneficial effects of argon plasma coagulation in the management of different types of gastric vascular ectasia lesions in patients admitted for GI hemorrhage. Gastrointestinal Endoscopy. 2008;**68**:440-446

[75] Smith LA, Morris AJ, Stanley AJ. The use of hemospray in portal hypertensive bleeding; a case series. Journal of Hepatology. European Association for the Study of the Liver. 2014;**60**:457-460

[76] Urata J, Yamashita Y, Tsuchigame T, et al. The effects of transjugular intrahepatic portosystemic shunt on portal hypertensive gastropathy. Journal of Gastroenterology & Hepatology. 1998;**13**:1061-1067

[77] Ripoll C, Garcia-Tsao G. The management of portal hypertensive gastropathy and gastric antral vascular ectasia. Digestive and Liver Disease. 2011;**43**:345-351

[78] Helton WS, Maves R, Wicks K, Johansen K. Transjugular intrahepatic portosystemic shunt vs surgical shunt in good-risk cirrhotic patients: A case-control comparison. Archives of Surgery. 2001;**136**:17-20

[79] Qureshi K, Al-Osaimi AM. Approach to the management of portal hypertensive gastropathy and gastric antral vascular ectasia. Gastroenterology Clinics of North America. 2014;**43**:835-847

Chapter 5

Portal Hypertensive Gastropathy (PHG)

Samia Ali Gamie

Additional information is available at the end of the chapter

http://dx.doi.org/10.5772/intechopen.69539

Abstract

Reversal of erosive gastritis in patients with portal hypertension by surgical shunts evolves the term of portal hypertensive gastropathy. In 1984, Sarfeh et al. addressed the term PHG to describe the distinctive erosive gastritis in patients with portal hypertension. Since that time, the recorded incidence of PHG in the studies has varied widely from 20 to 75% in patients with portal hypertension, with or without liver cirrhosis. As the underlying pathophysiology of the disease is unclear, not all the patients with portal hypertension developed PHG. Thus, portal hypertension cannot be the only factor for the development of PHG. Patients with PHG presented with either acute or chronic bleedings. Acute presentation is an emergency case. Anemia from chronic bleeding is a frequent presentation in PHG patients. The diagnosis is confirmed by a characteristic endoscopic appearance of PHG. Capsule endoscopy and dynamic CT are also used for the diagnosis of PHG. The goal of the treatment of PHG is reducing the portal pressure in patients with acute or chronic bleeding. Pharmacological treatment, endoscopic therapy, trans-jugular intrahepatic portosystemic shunt (TIPS), and shunt surgery are different modalities for treatment of PHG. Yet, primary prophylaxis treatment is not recommended in the patients with PHG.

Keywords: portal hypertensive gastropathy, portal hypertension, gastropathy, GAVE, liver cirrhosis

1. Introduction

1.1. Definition

Portal hypertensive gastropathy (PHG) is a painless condition of gastric mucosal ectasia and impaired mucosal defense, typically seen in patients with portal hypertension [1].

Portal hypertension (PH) exists when the hydrostatic pressure in the portal vein or its branches has increased. Two important factors are implicated; vascular resistance and blood flow, thus if the pressure gradient anywhere along the portal venous system (between the portal vein, and hepatic veins or the inferior vena cava (IVC)) is increased, portal hypertension develops.

The normal portal venous pressure ranges from 5 to 10 mm Hg, therefore, if the hepatic venous pressure gradient (HVPG) is ≥10 mm Hg, significant portal hypertension is considered, but if the HVPG is ≥12 mm Hg, severe portal hypertension is diagnosed [2].

The causes of portal hypertension are classified into three categories related to anatomical consideration. First, are causes originating in the portal venous system before it reaches the liver (pre-hepatic), e.g. portal vein thrombosis, schistosomiasis, primary biliary cholangitis/primary sclerosing cholangitis, or congenital hepatic fibrosis. Second, are causes within the liver (intrahepatic) e.g. cirrhosis as a result of viral, non alcoholic fatty liver disease (NAFLD), or autoimmune. Finally, are causes between the liver and the heart (post-hepatic) e.g. Budd-Chiari syndrome, inferior vena cava obstruction, or hepatic veno-occlusive disease (**Table 1**). The most common cause of PH is cirrhosis [3].

1.2. Essentials to diagnose PHG

- Portal hypertension with or without cirrhosis.
- Characteristic endoscopic findings.

Prehepatic	Hepatic	Posthepatic
Portal vein thrombosis	Cirrhosis of any cause, e.g. chronic viral hepatitis, alcoholic, autoimmune, NAFLD, biliary atresia, etc.	Inferior vena cava obstruction
Arteriovenous fistula	Primary biliary cholangitis	Hepatic vein thrombosis
Splenomegaly	Primary sclerosing cholangitis	Budd-Chiari syndrome
	Schistosomiasis	Right sided heart failure, e.g. from constrictive pericarditis
	Congenital hepatic fibrosis	
	Nodular regeneration hyperplasia	
	Granulomatous or infiltrative diseases (Gaucher, sarcoidosis, amyloid deposition	
	Toxicity (from arsenic, copper, methotrexate, amiodarone, ...)	
	Veno-occlusive disease	

NAFLD, non alcoholic fatty liver disease.

Table 1. Condition associated with portal hypertension.

2. History

In 1984, Sarfeh et al. recognized a distinct form of gastric mucosal hemorrhage in patients who had portal hypertension, they called it "portal hypertensive gastritis". They reported that this mucosal lesion in patients with portal hypertension was reversed after the portacaval shunt, in contrary to the mucosal lesion of patients without portal hypertension. Therefore, they concluded that there is a unique mucosal change excited with portal hypertension. 1 year later, it was discovered that this mucosal change was not a form of gastritis as there is no evidence of inflammation in the mucosa. Specific histopathological findings described this change, and the term "portal hypertensive gastropathy" was introduced by McCormack et al. in 1985 as a separate entity. However, there was no grading system of the endoscopic findings to put an accurate score for this condition. Several grading systems like the three- category system, and the two-category system have been proposed in 1994. The clinical importance of grading classification system resides in the fact that patients with severe PHG have a higher chance to bleed than patients with mild PHG [4].

The overall mortality from gastrointestinal bleeding is up to 25% of the mortality in patients with cirrhosis. In recent years however, PHG has been recognized as a distinct entity of gastrointestinal bleeding in patients with cirrhosis and portal hypertension. While variceal hemorrhage and peptic ulcer disease are known as significant causes of GI bleeding in cirrhosis, PHG and gastric antral vascular ectasia (GAVE) should also be considered as important causes. However, PHG should be differentiated from GAVE, GAVE occurs in patients with cirrhosis and portal hypertension, in addition to other conditions, such as chronic renal failure, connective tissue disorders, and bone marrow transplantation. On the other hand, PHG occurs only in patients with portal hypertension, whether with or without cirrhosis. In patients with cirrhosis, PHG is more common than GAVE [5].

However, although the endoscopic, histological and hemodynamic features of PHG mucosa have been extensively studied, the pathogenesis of PHG is still poorly understood, its natural history is not clearly documented and its treatment needs to be improved [6].

3. Epidemiology

The incidence of PHG varies greatly, it ranges between 20 and 75% of patients with portal hypertension, of those, approximately 65–90% have mild PHG, whereas 10–25% have severe PHG. This wide discrepancy in results may be attributed to the fact that the study was carried out on different groups of patients; patients with cirrhosis, patients without cirrhosis, patients with different Child-Pugh score of liver failure, and lastly patients with history of previous esophageal eradication therapy [7]. It was noticed that higher prevalence of PHG is found in patients with severe portal hypertension, advanced liver disease, and post-eradication therapy of esophageal varices [8]. Conversely, the incidence of acute gastrointestinal bleeding (hematemesis and/or melena) in PHG patients with cirrhosis were low; reported incidences ranged from 2.5 to 30%, with the greatest occurrences being observed in patients with severe PHG [9].

On the other hand, PHG as a marker of portal hypertension has conflicting results among the studies. Its sensitivity, positive predictive value (PPV) and negative predictive value (NPV), vary considerably between the studies, but its specificity has been reported to be above 95%. Snake-skin pattern has higher specificity (93–100%) for the diagnosis of PHG [10].

PHG can present at any age, including pediatric or adult patients [7].

4. Pathophysiology

The pathogenesis of PHG is still poorly understood. Portal hypertension is essential in the presence of PHG, due to the mechanical effect of the increased pressure in the portal vein which leads to hyper-dynamic congestion with a net increase in the gastric blood flow, this increase occurs in the submucosal, muscle, and serosal layers, while decreasing in the mucosal layer due to congestion and stasis. These hemodynamic changes impair gastric mucosal defense mechanisms, which lead to release of pro-inflammatory mediators, and alter the growth factors which render gastric mucosa more susceptible to injury, and impair mucosal healing. This defenseless mucosa may explain the increase in the rate of bleeding from PHG, additionally this abnormal gastric microcirculation, may render gastric mucosa more vulnerable to hypoxia, and more susceptible to noxious gastric factors, such as aspirin and ethanol [4].

Many other factors have also been implicated in the pathogenesis of PHG such as increased production of nitric oxide (NO), oxygen free radicals, endothelin-1, tumor necrosis factor-α, and prostaglandins. The most important factor, NO, is a potent vasodilator secreted by endothelial cells which may underlie the gastric vascular dilation and hyper-dynamic circulation in PHG. Furthermore, the expression of transforming growth factor α (TGF-α) and the epidermal growth factor (EGF) receptors in the gastric mucosa were reported to be highly elevated in areas of spontaneous gastric injury. Recently, studies found other factors, like p53-upregulated modulator of apoptosis (PUMA), to be markedly induced in the gastric mucosa of PHG patients [11]. Increased gastric mucosal apoptosis and decreased mucosal proliferation, were also noted in rats with PGH.

5. Factors influencing the development of portal hypertensive gastropathy

Many factors related to portal hypertension affect the presence and the severity of PHG. As the commonest cause of portal hypertension is liver cirrhosis, the presence or absence of cirrhosis, and its severity, may also affect the PHG.

5.1. Factors related to portal hypertension

- **Severity of portal hypertension:** The frequency of PHG is strongly correlated with the severity of portal hypertension, as indicated by hepatic venous pressure gradient (HVPG), esophageal intra-variceal pressure, and/or presence of esophageal varices and its size [12]. It was also found that portal hypertension associates with severe PHG, but not mild PHG, this was evident in patients with severe PHG, which were discovered to have elevated HVPG, high hepatic sinusoidal resistance, and low hepatic blood flow, all markers of severe portal hypertension [12].

This leads us to the conclusion that not all patients with portal hypertension exhibit evidence of, or develop PHG. On the other hand, resolution of PHG, which occurs after intervention to decrease portal hypertension (by pharmacotherapy, trans-jugular intrahepatic portosystemic shunt (TIPS), or liver transplantation), may suggest an association between PHG and portal hypertension [13].

Thus, although PHG cannot be diagnosed without portal hypertension, it is however not the only factor that evokes PHG.

- **Correlation with varices**: Severe PHG is more common in patients with esophageal varices than patients without varices. It also, correlated positively with the size of varices; denoting, it was higher in those with large varices than in those with medium-sized or small varices [12].
- **Location of varices:** PHG was more commonly seen in patients with coexisting gastric and esophageal varices than in patients with only esophageal varices. Additionally, moderate or severe PHG was noted to be higher (not to a significant level) in patients with common collateral circulation *vs* uncommon collaterals. Portosystemic common collateral circulation includes esophageal varices, gastric varices, and vein dilatation (whether abdominal, umbilical, or hemorrhoid), while uncommon collaterals include splenorenal, gastric, renal, retroperitoneal, or cardiac angle venous shunts [14].
- **Portal vein diameter:** It was proposed that PHG is promoted by minimal collateral circulation since significant collaterals would otherwise reduce portal hypertension and gastric mucosal congestion. Later on, it was found that portal vein diameter in cirrhotic patients with PHG and no esophageal varices is greater than the portal vein diameter in patients with esophageal varices. This concept was further supported by the finding that patients with portal vein diameter < 12 mm have a significantly higher prevalence of esophageal varices than patients with larger portal vein diameter. It was then believed that the absence of reversed blood flow in the portal vein (due to the absence of hepatofugal flow), in patients without esophageal varices, meant that the pressure in the portal vein was not affected [15].
- **Esophageal variceal eradication:** PHG may appear for the first time in patients with portal hypertension, or increase in severity in patients with pre-exciting PHG after eradication of esophageal varices by either endoscopic variceal ligation or endoscopic variceal sclerotherapy [16], thus patients with well developed fundal varices are more liable to develop PHG after obliteration of the varices than patients with poorly developed fundal varices. Since fundal varices are usually formed by a gastro-renal shunt, this finding supports the view that the presence of a gastro-renal shunt may play a protective role in the development of PHG after variceal obliteration. Therefore; some patients may exhibit minimum or no change in PHG after esophageal eradication [17].

Other techniques are also used for obliteration of the esophageal varices including angiographic variceal obliteration (which increases the PHG frequency), and percutaneous transhepatic variceal embolization; after which 38% of the patients develop *De-novo* PHG. The development of PHG for the first time or its increase in frequency and/or its severity is attributed to increased gastric mucosal congestion due to a decrease in the blood flow in the esophageal varices, which leads to an increase in the portal blood flow.

This phenomenon can be explained by obliteration of the blood flow after eradication of esophageal varices, this can lead to increased portal pressure and redistribution of residual blood flow that had passed through the previously patent varices. This mechanism is supported by the finding that gastric mucosal blood flow increases after variceal ligation [4].

Some investigators believe that the higher rate of PHG in patients undergoing endoscopic variceal eradication (sclerotherapy or banding) merely reflects other factors rather than the procedures *per se*, factors like; increased duration of portal hypertension, advanced liver disease, or severe portal hypertension in patients selected to undergo variceal eradication, must be evaluated in patients who developed PHG or showed an increase in its severity [18]. Nevertheless, higher frequency of PHG in patients undergoing sclerotherapy, suggest that portal hypertension is still the main underlying cause of PHG

5.2. Factors related to liver cirrhosis

- **Cirrhotic vs non-cirrhotic portal hypertension:** Primary liver disease usually occurs in PHG, but is not essential for PHG, provided another cause of portal hypertension exists. Consequently, PHG can occur in patients with other causes of portal hypertension; non-cirrhotic portal fibrosis, pre-hepatic or post-hepatic portal hypertension [19].

  Portal pressure is not the only factor that is determinant of PHG, other factors, like cirrhosis, may be implicated in the development of the mucosal lesions, which are characteristic of PHG. PHG was found to occur more commonly in patients with cirrhotic liver than in non-cirrhotic portal hypertension patients, also the patients with cirrhosis have a more aggressive course of PHG with faster progression to more severe PHG as time advances [19].

Taking this in consideration, other factors may also be involved in the pathogenesis of PHG. For example, in patients with portal hypertension and cirrhosis, there is an increase in the level of many vasodilator substances in systemic circulation e.g. gastrin, secretin, and VIP, this increase in the level of vasodilator or the decrease in the sensitivity to vasoconstrictor substance may have a role in the underlying mechanism of PHG [10]. However, these changes were also found in cirrhotic patients not suffering from PHG, thus the exact picture of the pathogenesis is not yet fully understood.

- **Duration of liver disease:** The duration of liver disease positively correlates with development of PHG, with average cumulative incidence of 3% at 1 year, 10% at 2 years, and 24% at 3 years [7].

- **Liver disease severity:** PHG is correlated with liver disease severity, as measured by Child-Turcotte-Pugh score (CTP score) (**Table 2**), Child-Pugh stage C cirrhosis is associated with more frequent and faster progression of PHG. Also, it was found that cirrhotic patients with severe PHG (especially those without esophageal varices) had more frequent CTP stage C than patients with mild PHG [7].

Model for end-stage liver disease (MELD) is another important scoring system for assessing liver disease severity, which was found to significantly correlate with PHG severity [20].

On the other hand, the severity of PHG was correlated to markers of advanced liver disease (like hypoalbuminemia and hyperbilirubinemia) which are biochemical markers of advanced liver disease. Markers of portal hypertension (thrombocytopenia) and of insulin resistance (hyperglycemia), were also significant independent predictors of PHG [21].

5.3. Other factors

Many other factors may be involved in the pathogenesis of PHG, this includes thrombocytopenia or splenomegaly which are associated with the severity of PHG. Additional factors like an increase in the thickness of the lesser omentum and the presence of a splenorenal shunt were found to correlate with PHG in patients with chronic liver disease [22].

5.3.1. Factors that do not affect the risk of PHG

Although, portal hypertension is essential for PHG diagnosis, there is still no association between the etiology of portal hypertension and PHG. Similarly, as cirrhosis is the common cause of portal hypertension, there is no correlation between the underlying causes of cirrhosis and PHG. Moreover, in cirrhotic patients, the role of Helicobacter pylori (H. pylori) in the pathogenesis of PHG is not fully understood. Some contributed that Helicobacter has no role in the pathogenesis of PHG in these patients [23]. However, there is evidence of association between H. pylori infection and PHG in cirrhotic patients, in these patients, Helicobacter infection may be related to the severity of PHG. This was strengthened by the fact that there was mild improvement of PHG after H. pylori eradication. Therefore, we can conclude that there may be a minor role for H. pylori in the pathogenesis of PHG in cirrhotic patients [23]. Further studies on large number of patients are conducted to show the effect of H. pylori eradication in the treatment of PHG, especially severe portal gastropathy in cirrhosis.

Parameter	**Point assigned**		
	1	**2**	**3**
Albumin (g/dl)	>3.5	2.8–3.5	<2.8
Bilirubin (mg/dl)	<2	2–3	>3
INR	<1.7	1.7–2.3	>2.3
Ascites	None	Slight-moderate	Tense
Encephalopathy	0	1–2	3–4

A total Child-Turcotte-Pugh score of 5–6 considered class A, 7–9 is class B, and 10– 15 is class C. INR, international normalized ratio.

Table 2. Child-Turcotte-Pugh score.

Also, there is no evidence that there is any increase in the prevalence or severity of PHG with the use of either nonsteroidal anti-inflammatory drugs (NSAIDs), or COX-(cyclooxygenase)-2 inhibitor [24]. Another negative correlation was found between alcohol and smoking alongside PHG, thus there is no benefit from abstinence or quitting smoking [25]. Likewise, the presence of PHG was independent of patient's age, or sex.

6. Whom should go for screening for PHG

Patients with portal hypertension and chronic iron deficiency anemia who are suspected to have chronic bleeding should go for PHG screening. Chronic bleeding is diagnosed when there is either decrease in hemoglobin level below 2 g/dL within 6-month, or if there is presence of iron deficiency anemia with a positive fecal occult blood test. For those patients, upper endoscopy can confirm the diagnosis of PHG [26].

7. Natural history

PHG may change in an individual patient over time, about 30% of the patients with cirrhosis and mild PHG, progress to severe PHG during a 10 year follow up period, considering that these patients did not receive any prophylactic treatment. Most of the patients with worsening PHG, severe lesions, or *de novo* PHG develop bleeding. There are only a few improved cases in PHG without treatment [27]. Furthermore, Patients who have PHG associated with cirrhosis-related portal hypertension have more frequently persistent and progressive PHG, which is more likely to bleed than patients with PHG related to non-cirrhotic portal hypertension [9].

Although, as mentioned above, patients with previous endoscopic therapy (sclerotherapy or endoscopic variceal ligation) have a higher prevalence of PHG, the clinical course of PHG in this context, particularly in non cirrhotic portal hypertension, may be milder and transient [28].

PHG is a dynamic condition emphasized by the observation that 30% of patients who have endoscopic features of PHG remained unchanged throughout follow-up period, whereas 25% of patients show either worsening or improvement of the condition during the follow up period. Thus, not only can PHG appear for the first time or progress from mild to severe condition over time, but it can also revert from severe to mild, and even disappear completely with treatment [23].

8. Clinical picture

Most patients with PHG are asymptomatic, but a significant number of patients exhibit symptoms related to iron deficiency anemia from chronic GI bleeding. Bleeding from PHG may be either chronic occult blood in the stool, or overt which occurs in a smaller proportion of patients. Endoscopic diagnosis of acute hemorrhage from PHG is established when there is active bleeding from gastropathy lesions, if non-removable clots overlying these lesions is observed, or when there is PHG and no other cause of acute bleeding can be demonstrated after thorough evaluation of the gastrointestinal tract [9]. Recurrent bleeding is common in PHG after the initial episode.

Although all PHG patients with chronic bleeding develop severe chronic iron deficiency anemia, no study has evaluated the prevalence of PHG in cirrhotic patients with chronic iron deficiency anemia. In patients with portal hypertension, with or without cirrhosis and chronic iron deficiency anemia, chronic bleeding from PHG must be suspected, its diagnosis is confirmed by upper endoscopy. Comprehensive study of the whole gastrointestinal tract in these patients by capsule endoscopy is mandatory to exclude similar lesion elsewhere along gastrointestinal tract e.g. colonopathy [27].

8.1. Diagnosis

The diagnosis of PHG is done mainly by upper endoscopy. The endoscopic findings of PHG diagnosis was classified by the New Italian Endoscopic Club according to its severity based on the presence of four elementary lesions: mosaic like pattern, red point lesions, cherry red spots, and black brown spots (**Figure 1**) [29]. Early change in PHG is called scarletina, which appears as a fine pink speckling. On the other side, severe PHG appear as cherry red spots that may become confluent and is very friable, so it can actively bleed during endoscopy. These lesions are present predominantly in the fundus and/or the corpus of the stomach, yet PHG–like lesions have been described in other sites in the gastrointestinal tract e.g. the rectum, colon, and small bowel in asymptomatic patients and in patients with bleeding [29].

8.2. Endoscopic evaluation of PHG

The elementary lesions of PHG according to the New Italian Endoscopic Club for the Study and Therapy of Esophageal Varices [NIEC] classification are as follows [30]:

(1) Mosaic-like pattern (MLP); it is described as the presence of small, polygonal areas in the center (areola) surrounded by a whitish-yellow depressed border. The term mosaic is further subdivided according to the color of the areola into; mild, when the areola is uniformly pink, moderate, if the center is red, and severe, when the areola is uniformly red.

(2) Red-point lesions (RPLs) are defined as red, small, flat lesions, and <1 mm in size.

(3) Cherry-red spots (CRSs) are defined as red, round lesions, >2 mm in diameter, which slightly protrude into the lumen of the stomach.

(4) Black-brown spots (BBSs) are defined as irregularly flat spots, either black or brown in color, does not disappear after washing, and it is due to intra-mucosal hemorrhage.

PHG is classified by endoscopy, into mild, moderate and severe forms. PHG mucosa can be seen as snakeskin (MLP) in mild cases, while RPLs, CRSs or BBCs that is liable to bleeding, are found in severe cases, however, the presence of red or brown spots without bleeding is considered a moderate disease [35].

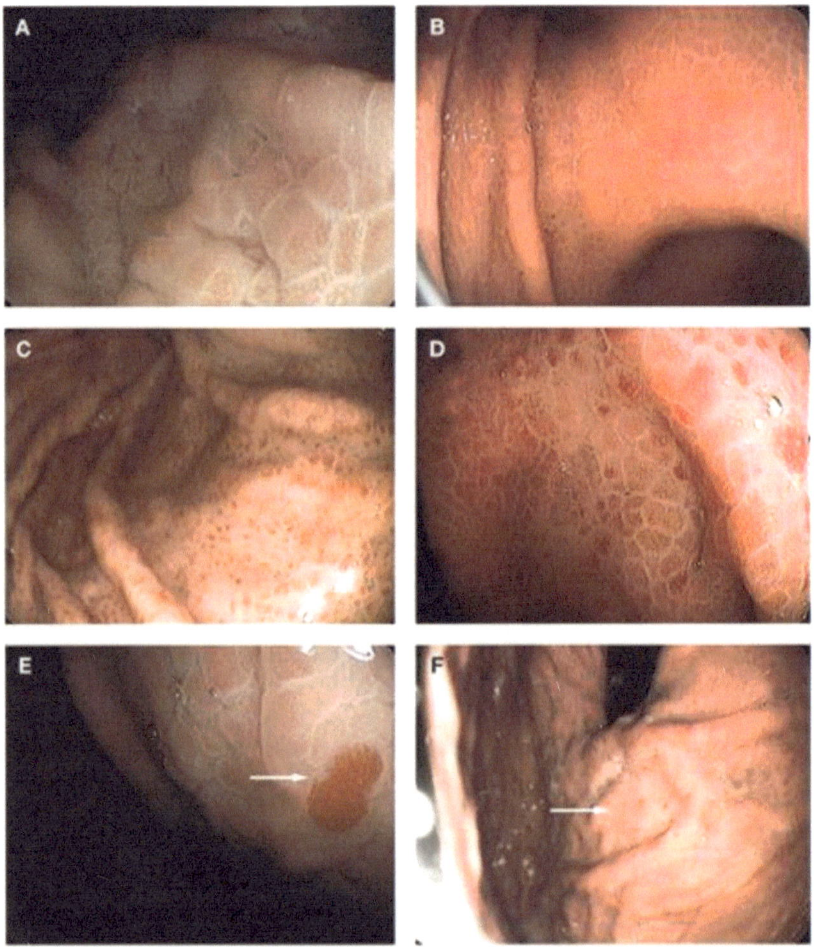

Figure 1. Endoscopic images of portal hypertensive gastropathy that show the four main findings of this condition. Mild (A) and moderate (B) mosaic-like gastric mucosal pattern, red point lesions (C), cherry-red spots (D), and black–brown spots, including an intramucosal hemorrhage (E) and a brown spot (F).

8.3. Classification of portal hypertensive gastropathy

PHG is classified on the basis of the condition's severity, therefore many classifications of the PHG mucosa have been proposed. McCormack's classification, NIEC's and Tanoue's classifications are the most popular used classifications (**Table 3**). McCormack classified the mucosal changes into two main categories, mild and severe, on the other hand, the NIEC classification has three categories; mild, moderate and severe, and further subdivided the mosaic-like pattern into three groups [28]. Finally, the McCormack classification, a two-category classification system, is the recommended one. The classification comprises of:

Mild portal hypertensive gastropathy: Only one change in the stomach mucosa is present, that of appearance of mosaic or snakeskin pattern on it.

http://dx.doi.org/10.5772/intechopen.69539

	McCormack	NIEC	Tanoue
Mild	Scarlatina type rash		
	Snake skin	Pink in center mosaic	Mild redness
	Striped appearance		
Moderate	–	Flat red spots mosaic	Fine red speckling mosaic
Severe	Red spots	Diffusely red mosaic	Point bleeding
	Diffuse hemorrhagic lesions		

Table 3. Endoscopic finding and classification of PHG.

Severe portal hypertensive gastropathy: In addition to the mosaic or snakeskin pattern of the stomach mucosa; bulging, flat red or black-brown spots are seen. There also may be active bleeding.

In the rare instance where PHG cannot be clearly diagnosed on the basis of endoscopic appearance and location alone, biopsy for histology may prove useful [28].

8.4. Histologically

The unique histological features of PHG are marked dilatation of the capillaries and collecting venules in the gastric mucosa with markedly congested and tortuous submucosal venules (**Figure 2**) [31]. These vascular features are present in the absence of any inflammatory cell

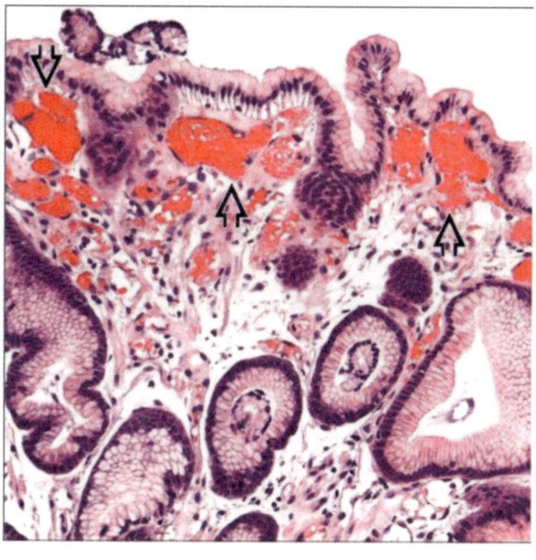

Figure 2. Hematoxylin and eosin shows numerous dilated capillaries in the superfacial gastric mucosa. These are not entirely specific for PHG.

infiltrate or erosion of the gastric mucosa. Stromal fibrosis and edema of the lamina propria can also be seen [31].

It may be difficult to differentiate between severe PHG and gastric antral vascular ectasia (GAVE) by endoscopic examination, so biopsy is beneficial in this case, as GAVE has distinct histological features that can set it apart from severe PHG. GAVE has many fibrin thrombi in the mucosal vessels with ectasia and spindle cell proliferation (smooth muscle and myofibroblast hyperplasia) in the superficial mucosa. Furthermore, fibrohyalinosis is more commonly present in GAVE. All of these findings provide additional features that help in differentiating between severe PHG and GAVE [32].

8.5. Portal gastropathy score calculation

Table 4 shows the scoring system to calculate the severity of PHG, the calculation depends on three categories: *Microscopic picture*; score 1 considered for mild findings, and score 2 for severe findings. *Red marks*; isolated lesion is considered score 1, whereas confluent red marks is scored 2. *GAVE*; if absent scored 0, while its presence is scored 2. If the total score was equal to 3 or less, the PHG is mild, on the other hand if the score is 4 or greater, PHG is severe [33].

8.6. Other diagnostic modalities

8.6.1. Non-endoscopic methods for diagnosis of HPG

Other non-endoscopic methods for the diagnosis of PHG such as MRI and CT are not yet considered as routine investigation for the diagnosis of PHG. Their results must be further evaluated to warrant their role in the diagnosis of PHG. Endoscopy still remains the main diagnostic method [34].

In CT scan, enhancement of the inner layer of the gastric walls due to gastric congestion, characterizes PHG lesion. Similarly, MRI is used to measure the diameter of collateral veins e.g. the left gastric, paraesophageal, and azygos veins to confirm the diagnosis of portal hypertension. In patients with PHG, the measurement of the diameters of these veins does not differ from those

Endoscopic findings	Parameter	Score
Mucosal mosaic pattern	Mild	1
	Severe	2
Red markings	Isolated	1
	Confluent	2
Gastric antral vascular ectasia (GAVE)	Absence	1
	Presence	2

Mild portal hypertensive gastropathy ≤ 3; severe portal hypertensive gastropathy ≥ 4.

Table 4. Portal hypertensive Gastropathy scoring system.

in patients without PHG, therefore it is not helpful in the diagnosis. These data suggest that these imaging techniques is still in its infancy period and best reserved for experimental purposes [35].

8.7. Differential diagnosis

The endoscopic findings of the gastric mucosa include many differential diagnoses of several disorders. When red spots are seen in the stomach by endoscopy, important diagnostic considerations are evoked. GAVE or watermelon stomach which is a common differential diagnosis of PHG, has characteristic endoscopic findings which are linear red stripes, separated by normal mucosa, these findings give the appearance of a watermelon, that is seen in the gastric antrum or proximal stomach. GAVE and PHG are distinct entities, however both are encountered in cirrhotic patients. While PHG routinely affects the gastric body and fundus, GAVE almost exclusively inhabits the antrum [32].

These findings have a diagnostic accuracy of 85% for GAVE and help distinguish it from PHG.

Table 5 further shows the differences between GAVE and PHG, however, there may be an overlap between GAVE and PHG in cirrhosis with portal hypertension [6].

Other conditions that increase the dilemma of PHG diagnosis include simple acute gastritis caused by non-steroidal anti–inflammatory drug (NSAIDS) or *H. pylori*, which may have a mosaic like pattern endoscopically but, the main histopathological feature in gastritis is inflammatory cell infiltration with minor vascular dilation, and it is also localized to the mucosa (superficial lesion). Lastly, endoscopic lesions similar to PHG may be also seen in some uncommon diseases e.g. polycythemia, gastric purpura, and Osler-Weber-Rendu disease [36].

	PHG	GAVE
Underlying etiology	Portal hypertension with or without cirrhosis	Can be present without portal hypertension, such as chronic renal failure, connective tissue disorders, and bone marrow transplantation
Predominant location	Fundus and corpus	Antrum
Endoscopic appearance	Mosaic like pattern or red marks	Linear red strips separated by normal mucosa
Pathological findings	Dilatation of the capillaries, and collecting venules in the gastric mucosa. Ectasia of submucosal veins, with intimal thickening	Fibrin microthrombi, myofibroplast hyperplasia, fibrinolysis
Management		
• **Response to beta blockers**	Yes	No
• **TIPS**	Yes	No
• **Endoscopic therapy ACP**	Used in refractory bleeding	Preferable as first line

ACP, argon plasma coagulation.

Table 5. Comparison between portal hypertensive gastropathy and gastric antral vascular ectasia.

9. Management of PHG

The goal of management of PHG is to reduce portal pressure.

9.1. Primary prophylaxis

PHG in asymptomatic patients who have no evidence of bleeding is discovered accidentally during screening for either chronic iron deficiency anemia or for esophageal varices in patients with cirrhosis. Till now, there is no recommendation to start any primary prophylaxis to prevent bleeding from PHG patients, except if there is an indication of beta-blocker for other reasons. However, in asymptomatic patients with both esophageal varices and PHG, if the patient undergoes esophageal eradication therapy, co-administration of a nonselective beta-blocker is beneficial. The dose of beta blocker should be titrated to a goal heart rate of 55–60 bpm or a 25% reduction from baseline. On the other hand, in patients with severe PHG and no varices, starting prophylaxis therapy with nonselective beta-blockers, should be considered. Yet, this approach is controversial, and more research is needed to clarify the prophylactic role of beta-blockers as primary prophylaxis for bleeding from PHG [34].

9.2. Secondary prophylaxis

Beta-blockers (like propranolol or nadolol) are used as secondary prophylaxis, and are the basis of therapy, to prevent recurrent bleeding from PHG. It is not only used to prevent the bleeding, but it also improves the severity score of PHG by endoscopy, changing it from severe to mild, or even completely curing it. On the other hand, about 50% of PHG patients especially cirrhotic during a 2-year follow up, show mild or even no response to beta blocker therapy. For those patients adding isosorbide 5-mononitrate may have a synergistic effect to reduce the portal pressure [37].

Addition of beta-blocker therapy to endoscopic management of varices is beneficial in reducing the progression of PHG after endoscopic therapy of varices. Propranolol, a non-selective beta-blocker (24–480 mg/day), has been commonly used in these cases. The dose of propranolol should be increased gradually to maximum dose (up to 160 mg twice daily) with targeted heart rate of 55–60 bpm, and should be continued as long as there is portal hypertension [37]. In patients with iron deficiency anemia, iron replacement therapy and beta blocker should be started simultaneously.

9.3. Treatment of chronic bleeding

Patients with PHG with or without cirrhosis, and chronic blood loss are commonly presented with iron deficiency anemia. Thorough investigation of these patients must be done to rule out other causes of iron deficiency anemia before attributing PHG as the cause. All patients with PHG and iron deficiency anemia should start iron-replacement therapy either; oral preparations, or intravenous (IV) iron.

To reduce chronic bleeding from PHG, with or without portal hypertension, portal pressure should be reduced, therefore non selective beta blocker is the first line of treatment. The use of beta blockers has proved efficient, based on both experimental and clinical investigations demonstrating that, propranolol reduces portal pressure and cause vasoconstriction in the overall splanchnic vascular bed.

Anti-oxidants have also been used to treat PHG. Experimentally, Vitamin E led to complete reversal of susceptibility of PHG mucosa to alcohol injury, in rats. Vitamin E also, led to the restoration of normal Extracellular signal-regulated kinase (ERK-2 signaling), which plays a pivotal role in healing after gastric mucosal injury. Thus, vitamin E may have a protective effect on the PHG mucosa [38].

Use of other pharmacological agents such as losartan, thalidomide and corticosteroids have been prescribed in the treatment of chronic bleeding from PHG. However, the evidence supporting their use in PHG bleeding is weak [39].

9.4. Treatment of acute bleeding

- For acute bleeding; initial stabilization with octreotide or terlipressin to stop the bleeding, followed by initiation of beta-blockers as secondary prevention is recommended. During acute bleeding from PHG, the patients may be hemodynamically unstable, therefore beta blocker therapy must be reserved, regarding its drawback, as it has a negative effect on heart and the circulation. Despite the drawbacks of beta-blocker therapy, it is considered immediately after the patient becomes hemodynamically stable, usually within 3 days. This highlights their important role in the management of acute as well as chronic GI bleeding.
- Octreotide, a somatostatin analogue (100 μg bolus followed by an infusion of 25 μg/h for 48 h), and Terlipressin, a vasopressin analogue, are both effective in the treatment of acute bleeding caused by PHG. Vasopressin and omeprazole when used together are more effective in controlling the acute bleeding than when vasopressin is used alone [40].

9.5. For refractory cases

When the patients do not respond to the previously mentioned treatments, invasive intervention must be done. Transjugular intrahepatic portosystemic shunt (TIPS) or surgical shunt are considered as salvage therapy only when they are performed in certain circumstances and in an expert center due to their significant morbidity and mortality results [41].

Surgical shunting has also proved beneficial in refractory bleeding from PHG however, this benefit is limited by an increase in the risk of deterioration of the hepatic function in patients with cirrhosis. Only cirrhotic patients with Child Pugh score A or B found improved outcomes from surgical shunting with reduced mortality. Comparing the results of TIPS with surgical shunt, it is reported that surgical shunt reduced re-bleeding, with fewer shunt complication e.g. shunt revisions, stent thrombosis, re-stenosis, and re-intervention of TIPS. However, long-term mortality was similar. On the other hand, similar results were found between TIPSS and distal splenorenal shunting with regards to re-bleeding, encephalopathy, and survival. Whatever the method of shunting in case of refractory bleeding from PHG, it should always be performed in expertise center. Surgical shunting may be an option only in CTP stage A cirrhosis with PHG or in patients with non-cirrhotic portal hypertension [42].

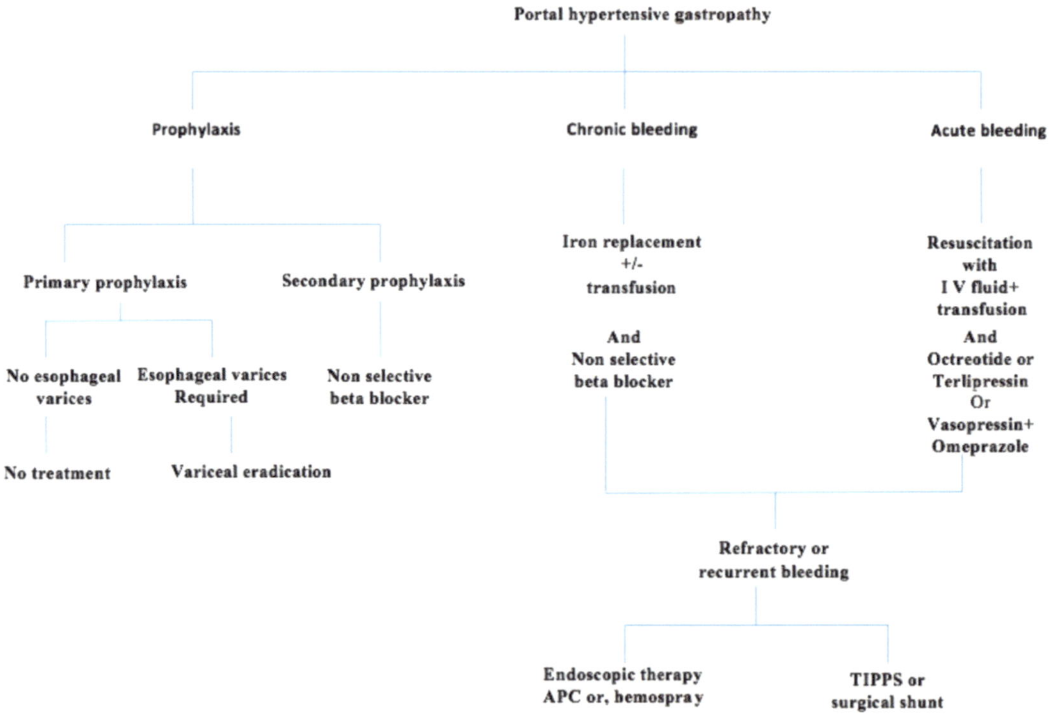

Figure 3. Treatment algorithm of portal hypertensive gastropathy.

Argon plasma coagulation (APC) is an electrosurgical technique used for treatment of bleeding of PHG. APC is a noncontact thermal coagulation, high frequency current, that is applied to the bleeding site through an argon plasma jet, this creates effective hemostasis and a homogenous surface coagulation with limited depth penetration. Treatment with APC decrease the need of transformation and improve the hemoglobin level in PHG patients, accordingly APC is an effective and rapid therapy to control bleeding from PHG, especially if there is a contraindication for beta blockers. If beta blocker can be used, co administration with APC has a synergistic effect in controlling PHG bleeding [5].

Hemospray: In patients with acute active bleeding due to PHG, it may be useful to use hemostatic powder that acts as a barrier to enhance the action of the clotting factors, giving time for the coagulation process to act and stop the bleeding [43]. A treatment algorithm for patients with PHG is described in **Figure 3**.

10. Mortality rates

Limited data on mortality due to bleeding from PHG is available, but the bleeding from PHG is rarely fatal. It represents a small percentage if compared with the mortality from other causes of gastrointestinal bleeding due to portal hypertension, and especially in comparison to variceal bleeding. Also, in cirrhotic patients it represents only <1% of the mortality, because the bleeding is typically mild [4]. As bleeding from PHG is an unusual direct cause of death, it does not affect the survival in cirrhotic patients. However, anemia from chronic bleeding or repeated acute bleeding may lead to deterioration of the liver function.

Acknowledgements

I would like to thank my family for their continuous support. Mohamed & Mennat Allah for the late nights they stayed up with me. To my husband Megahed and my daughter Reem, I'm grateful for them inspiring and pushing me to do this in the first place. I'm eternally grateful to all of you.

Author details

Samia Ali Gamie

Address all correspondence to: samia_ali5@hotmail.com

Faculty of Medicine, Helwan University, Cairo, Egypt

References

[1] Snyder P, Ali R, Poles M, Gross SA. Portal hypertensive gastropathy with a focus on management. Expert Review of Gastroenterology & Hepatology. 2015;**9**(9):1207-1216

[2] Bandali MF, Mirakhur A, Lee EW, Ferris MC, Sadler DJ, Gray RR, et al. Portal hypertension: Imaging of portosystemic collateral pathways and associated image-guided therapy. World Journal of Gastroenterology. 2017;**23**(10):1735-1746

[3] Bloom S, Kemp W. Portal hypertension: pathophysiology, diagnosis and management. Internal Medicine Journal. 2015;**45**(1):16-26

[4] Mihajlo GjeorgievskiAl, Cappell MS. Portal hypertensive gastropathy: A systematic review of the pathophysiology, clinical presentation, natural history and therapy. World Journal of Hepatology. 2016;**8**(4):231-262

[5] Amr Shaaban Hanafy, Amr Talaat El Hawary. Efficacy of argon plasma coagulation in the management of portal hypertensive gastropathy. Endoscopy International Open. 2016;**4**(10):E1057–E1062

[6] Patwardhan VR, Cardenas A. Review article: The management of portal hypertensive gastropathy and gastric antral vascular ectasia in cirrhosis. Alimentary Pharmacology & Therapeutics. 2014;**40**:354-362

[7] Merli M, Nicolini G, Angeloni S, Gentili F, Attili AF, Riggio O. The natural history of portal hypertensive gastropathy in patients with liver cirrhosis and mild portal hypertension The American Journal of Gastroenterology. 2004;**99**:1959-654

[8] Thuluvath PJ, Yoo HY. Portal hypertensive gastropathy. The American Journal of Gastroenterology. 2002;**97**:2973-2978

[9] Cristina Ripoll, Guadalupe Garcia-Tsao. Management of gastropathy and gastric vascular ectasia in portal hypertension. Clinical Liver Disease. 2010;**14**(2):281-295

[10] Eleftheriadis E. Portal hypertensive gastropathy a clinically significant puzzle. Annals of Gastroenterology. 2001;**14**(3):196-204

[11] Wang J, Han W, Zborowska E, Liang J, Wang X, Willson JK, Sun L, Brattain MG. Reduced expression of transforming growth factor beta type I receptor contributes to the malignancy of human colon carcinoma cells. The Journal of Biological Chemistry. 1996;**271**(29):17366-17371

[12] Abbasi A, Bhutto AR, Butt N, Munir SM, Dhillo AK. Frequency of portal hypertensive gastropathy and its relationship with biochemical, haematological and endoscopic features in cirrhosis. Journal of the College of Physicians and Surgeons Pakistan. 2011;**21**:723-726

[13] Kamath PS, Shah VH. Portal hypertension and bleeding esophageal varices. In: Boyer TD, Manns MP, Sanyal AJ, editors. In: Zakim and Boyer's Hepatology: A Textbook of Liver Disease. 6th ed. Philadelphia: Elsevier Saunders. 2012: pp. 296-326

[14] Wu Q, Shen L, Chu J, Ma X, Jin B, Meng F, Chen J, Wang Y, Wu L, Han J, et al. Characterization of uncommon portosystemic collateral circulations in patients with hepatic cirrhosis. Oncology Letters. 2015;**9**:347-350

[15] Zardi EM, Uwechie V, Gentilucci UV, Dobrina A, Petitti T, Laghi V, Picardi A, Afeltra A. Portal diameter in the diagnosis of esophageal varices in 266 cirrhotic patients: Which role? Ultrasound in Medicine & Biology. 2007;**33**:506-511

[16] Elnaser MS, Elebiary S, Bastawi MB, El Shafei A, Elmagd IM, Hamza MM. The prevalence of portal hypertensive gastropathy and duodenopathy in some Egyptian cirrhotic patients. Ultrasound in Medicine & Biology. 2004;**34**:915-923

[17] Iwao T, Toyonaga A, Oho K, et al. Portal-hypertensive gastropathy develops less in patients with cirrhosis and fundal varices. Journal of Hepatology. 1997;**26**:1235-1241

[18] Feldman M, Lee EL. Gastritis. In: Feldman M, Friedman LS, Brandt LJ, editors. Sleisenger and Fordtran's Gastrointestinal and Liver Disease: Pathophysiology, Diagnosis, Management. 10th ed. Philadelphia: Elsevier Saunders; 2010. pp. 868-883

[19] Sogaard KK, Astrup LB, Vilstrup H, Gronbaek H. Portal vein thrombosis; risk factors, clinical presentation and treatment. BMC Gastroenterology. 2007;**7**:34

[20] MY, Choi H, Baik SK, Yea CJ, Won CS, Byun JW, Park SY, Kwon YH, Kim JW, Kim HS, et al. Portal hypertensive gastropathy: Correlation with portal hypertension and prognosis in cirrhosis. Digestive Diseases and Sciences. 2010;**55**:3561-3567

[21] Zardi EM, Ghittoni G, Margiotta D, Viera FT, Di Matteo F, Rossi S. Portal hypertensive gastropathy in cirrhotics without varices: A case-control study. European Journal of Gastroenterology & Hepatology. 2015;**27**:91-96

[22] Kim MY, Choi H, Baik SK, Yea CJ, Won CS, Byun JW, Park SY, Kwon YH, Kim JW, Kim HS, et al. Portal hypertensive gastropathy: Correlation with portal hypertension and prognosis in cirrhosis. Digestive Diseases and Sciences. 2010;**55**:3561-3567

[23] Khaled Abd-Alazeim Eid, Muhammad Abd El-Gawad Shawky MD, Amro Metwaly Hassan, Ahmed Qasem Mohammed, Mostafa Ismail Mohammed. Prevalence of *Helicobacter pylori* infection in patients with portal hypertensive gastropathy owing to liver cirrhosis Al-Azhar Assiut Medical Journal. 2016;**14**(3):109-114

[24] Fontana RJ, Sanyal AJ, Mehta S, Doherty MC, Neuschwander-Tetri BA, Everson GT, Kahn JA, Malet PF, Sheikh MY, Chung RT, et al. Portal hypertensive gastropathy in chronic hepatitis C patients with bridging fibrosis and compensated cirrhosis: results from the HALT-C trial. The American Journal of Gastroenterology. 2006;**101**:983-992

[25] Herbst DA, Reddy KR. Risk factors for hepatocellular carcinoma. Clinical Liver Disease. 2012;**1**(6):180-182. DOI: 10.1002/cld.111

[26] Sanyal AJG, Grace ND, Carey W. Prevention and management of gastroesophageal varices and variceal hemorrhage in cirrhosis. Hepatology. 2007;**46**:922-938

[27] Misra SP, Dwivedi M, Misra V. Prevalence and factors influencing hemorrhoids, anorectal varices, and colopathy in patients with portal hypertension. Endoscopy. 1996;**28**(4): 340-345

[28] D'Amico G, Garcia-Tsao G, Pagliaro L. Natural history and prognostic indicators of survival in cirrhosis: A systematic review of 118 studies. Journal of Hepatology. 2006;**44**: 217-231

[29] Rafael F Perini, Paula RS Camara and Jose GP Ferraz. Nature clinical practice, pathogenesis of portal hypertensive gastropathy: Translating basic research into clinical practice. Gastroenterology & Hepatology. 2009;**6**:150-158. DOI: 10.1038/ncpgasthep1356

[30] Spina GP, Arcidiacono R, Bosch J. et al. Gastric endoscopic features in portal hypertension: Final report of a consensus conference, Milan, Italy. 19 September 1992. 1994. pp. 461-467

[31] Amitabh Srivastava MD. Pathology & laboratory medicine, basicmedical insight engine. http://basicmedicalkey.com/portal-hypertensive-gastropathy [Accessed: July 6, 2016]

[32] Burak KW, Lee SS, Beck PL. Portal hypertensive gastropathy and gastric antral vascular ectasia (GAVE). Journal of Hepatology. 2001;**49**:866-872

[33] Charmaine Stewart A, Arun Sanyal J. Grading portal gastropathy: Validation of a gastropathy scoring system. The American Journal of Gastroenterology. 2003;**98**:1758-1765. DOI: 10.1111/j.1572-0241.2003.07595

[34] Urrunaga NH, Don Rockey C. Portal hypertensive gastropathy and colopathy. Clinical Liver Disease. 2014;**18**(2):389-406

[35] Erden A, Idilman R, Erden I, et al. Veins around the esophagus and the stomach: Do their calibrations provide a diagnostic clue for portal hypertensive gastropathy? Clinical Imaging. 2009;**33**:22-24

[36] Raul Cubillas, Don Rockey C. Portal hypertensive gastropathy: A review article. Liver International . 2010;**30**(8):1094-1102. DOI: 10.1111/j.1478-3231.2010.02286

[37] Lo GH, Lai KH, Cheng JS, Hsu PI, Chen TA, Wang EM, Lin CK, Chiang HT. The effects of endoscopic variceal ligation and propranolol on portal hypertensive gastropathy: A prospective, controlled trial. Gastrointestinal Endoscopy. 2001;**53**:579-584

[38] Thuluvath PJ, Yoo HY. Portal hypertensive gastropathy. The American Journal of Gastroenterology. 2002;**97**:2973-2978

[39] Wagatsuma Y, Naritaka Y, Shimakawa T. et al. Clinical usefulness of the angiotensin II receptor antagonist losartan in patients with portal hypertensive gastropathy. Hepatogastroenterology. 2006;**53**(68):171-174

[40] Zhou Y, Qiao L, Wu J. et al. Comparison of the efficacy of octreotide, vasopressin, and omeprazole in the control of acute bleeding in patients with portal hypertensive gastropathy: A controlled study. Journal of Gastroenterology and Hepatology. 2002;**17**:973-979

[41] Kamath PS, Lacerda M, Ahlquist DA, McKusick MA, Andrews JC, Nagorney DA. Gastric mucosal responses to intrahepatic portosystemic shunting in patients with cirrhosis. Gastroenterology. 2000;**118**:905-911

[42] De Franchis R, Faculty BV. Revising consensus in portal hypertension: report of the Baveno V consensus workshop on methodology of diagnosis and therapy in portal hypertension. Journal of Hepatology. 2010;**53**:762-768

[43] Smith LA, Morris AJ, Stanley AJ. The use of hemospray in portal hypertensive bleeding; A case series. European association for the study of the liver. Journal of Hepatology. 2014;**60**:457-460

Chapter 6

Application of Transmission Electron Microscopy Techniques in the Veterinary Diagnosis of Viral Gastroenteritis in Livestock Animals

Marcia Helena Braga Catroxo and
Ana Maria Cristina Rebello Pinto da Fonseca Martins

Additional information is available at the end of the chapter

http://dx.doi.org/10.5772/intechopen.70945

Abstract

Gastroenteritis caused by viruses is considered to be one of the most important diseases in livestock, being the main cause of morbidity and mortality in young animals, culminating in serious economic losses due to costs with prophylaxis and treatment, increased susceptibility of animals to secondary infections, developmental delay and death. Stressful factors may support the onset of illness. Several viral agents can cause gastroenteritis in various animal species. Rotaviruses are considered the main cause of enteric infections in various animals, including humans constituting important zoonosis. Due to genetic diversity and their ability to cross the species barrier, the coronaviruses infect many species. In cattle, they cause "Winter Dysentery" in adult animals and "Neonatal Diarrhea" in newborn calves. In swine, they are responsible for "Transmissible Gastroenteritis" and "Swine Epidemic Diarrhea." Equines infected with coronavirus also develop severe gastroenteritis. Bovine viral diarrhea (BVD) caused by a flavivirus of the genus *Pestivirus* is related to digestive and reproductive disorders, affecting any productive sector, are it cut, milk or confinement. Transmission electron microscopy is an indispensable tool in the diagnosis of viral gastroenteric infectious diseases. Negative staining is a simple, fast and efficient technique, being ideal for the detection of gastroenteric viruses, being easily visualized. The immunoelectron microscopy (IEM) technique allows increasing the sensitivity of virus detection where low concentrations of virus are aggregated so that they may be more easily seen. The immunolabeling with colloidal gold technique utilizes specific antibodies tagged with particles of colloidal gold to label the antigen antibody reaction. Embedding resin technique allows obtaining information on the virus–cell interaction. The different transmission electron microscopy modalities promotes a fast and accurate diagnosis of the different gastroenteric viral agents, allowing prophylactic measures of control and prevention in the creations to be promptly instituted, avoiding animal losses and disastrous economic losses, and collaborating with the National Porcine and Bovine Agribusiness.

Keywords: viral gastroenteritis, livestock animals, veterinary diagnostic, transmission electron microscopy

1. Introduction

Gastroenteritis caused by viruses is considered one of the most important diseases in livestock, being the main cause of morbidity and mortality in neonates. The food animal livestock industry estimated a multimillion dollar annual economic loss due to diarrheal diseases associated with a reduction in weight gain, costs with prophylaxis and treatment, increased susceptibility of animals to secondary infections, developmental delay and death of young animals. They represent an important sanitary problem compromising the herds, independently of the level of technification of the creation. Stressful factors such as long-distance travel, reproduction, nutritional deficiencies, environmental changes, etc., may support the onset of illness [1].

The main agents that can cause gastroenteritis in livestock animals are rotavirus, coronavirus and flavivirus.

1.1. Rotavirus

Rotaviruses are considered the main cause of enteric infections in cattle, swine, equines, canines, felines, birds and wild, including humans constituting important zoonosis [2, 3]. They are observed more frequently in neonates, with negative economic impact to the worldwide productive sector, causing high mortality, when it occurs in commercial creations. In livestock, rotaviruses are associated with severe enteric diseases in young calves [4, 5], weaning and postweaning piglets [6] and severe enteritis in foals [7].

Rotavirus is classified as a member of *Reoviridae* family, *Sedovirinae* subfamily and *Rotavirus* genus [8]. They have icosahedral symmetry and a nonenveloped capsid formed by three concentric layers of protein that is 70–90 in diameter. The genome of rotavirus comprises 11 segments of double-strand RNA of 16–21 kbp, encoding six structural proteins (VP1–VP4, VP6 and VP7) and five nonstructural proteins (NSp1–NSp5/6). They are classified into eight groups (A–H) based on the antigenic relationship of its VP6 protein. The most common groups that infect humans and animals are the A, B and C [9, 10].

1.1.1. Bovine rotavirus

Bovine group A rotavirus (bovine RVA) is recognized as the most common cause of severe gastroenteritis in cattle, causing significant economic loss in the dairy and beef industry due to increased morbidity and mortality, treatment costs and reduced growth rates [11, 12].

http://dx.doi.org/10.5772/intechopen.70945

Infection with bovine rotavirus group A (RVA) has been reported in several countries, such as Brazil [12], the Netherlands [13], Australia [14], EUA [15], New Zealand [16] and Japan [17]. Rotavirus B strains also cause epidemic and sporadic cases of diarrhea in humans, pigs, cattle, limbs and rats [18]. Bovine RVB infections have been reported only in Japan [19], Indian [20], the United Kingdom [21] and the United States [22].

Rotaviral diarrhea usually affects calves between 4 days and 3 weeks old. The incubation period is 12–24 h, and the duration of diarrhea lasts from 2 to 5 days [19, 23–25].

The animals presented depression, anorexia, excessive salivation, profuse diarrhea and severe dehydration [23, 24]. The abomasums typically contains milk curd and thick saliva. The virus replicates in the mature epithelial cells of the villi, and viral infection redirects the function of cells of the absorption for the partially digested milk and accumulates in the intestinal lumen [24, 26]. Other secondary agents often found in epizootics of rotavirus-associated diarrhea may contribute to the severity of the disease [26].

Transmission generally occurs when an unaffected animal has oral contact with infected feces and contaminated feed, or if they are exposed to living quarters with poor hygiene characteristics. Cows displaying signs and symptoms may shed the virus for as long as a week, while some cows can become reinfected and shed the virus throughout their life and remain asymptomatic [26].

The methods of negative staining (rapid preparation) (**Figure 1**) and the immunoelectron microscopy (**Figure 2**) demonstrate the presence of rotavirus particles in fecal samples from calves with diarrhea [25], being named "the gold standard" in the diagnosis of viral enteritis in calves. Immune electron microscopy (**Figure 2**) and immunolabeling with colloidal gold particles (**Figure 3**) have a high sensitivity ranging from 87 to 100% of the different viral agents, which gives good diagnostic value [27, 28].

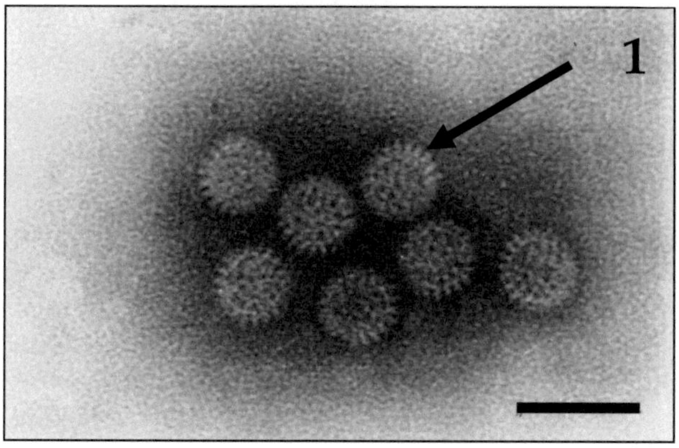

Figure 1. Negatively-stained rotavirus particles, showing individual capsomers (arrow) in feces of bovine. Bar: 80 nm.

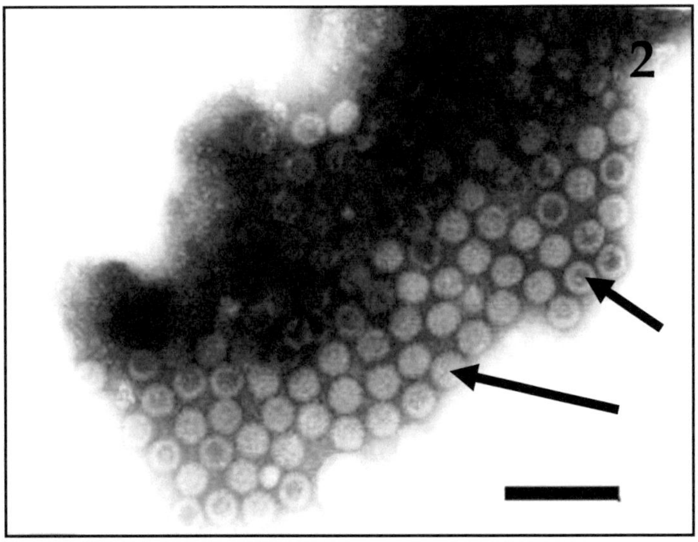

Figure 2. Immunoelectron microscopy of rotavirus particles aggregated by antigen–antibody interaction in bovine feces. Observe "complete" (big arrow) and "empty" (minor arrow) particles. Bar: 240 nm.

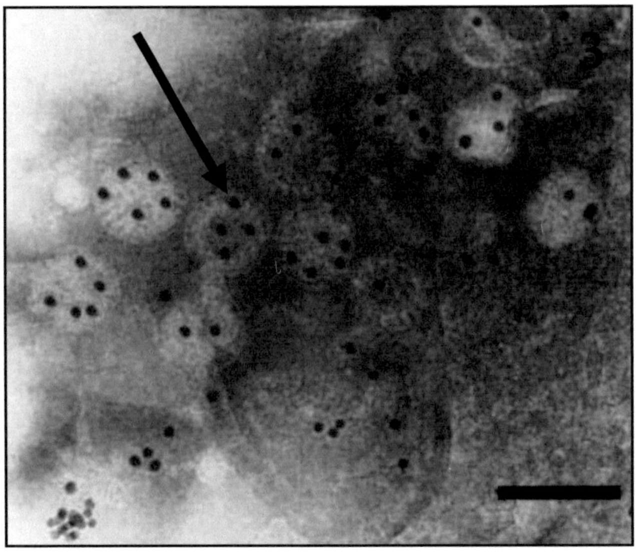

Figure 3. Bovine rotavirus marked by the particles of colloidal gold (arrow). Bar: 100 nm.

General recommendations regarding decrease of RVA diarrhea include management practices, especially good hygiene and sanitation procedures, as well as pathogen-specific interventions, such as the use of vaccine prophylaxis [14, 29].

1.1.2. *Swine rotavirus*

In pig farms, rotaviruses are responsible for economic losses due to death of animals, poor growth performance and costs of diagnostic and treatment [30, 31].

The rotaviruses that affect pigs are differentiated as group A, B and C, based on the antigenicity and genetic characteristics of VP6 [9, 32]. Group H has already been described in Brazil [33]. Group A rotavirus is the most frequently isolated of piglets with 1- to 8-week-old diarrhea [34], but groups B and C are also described in piglets in both the maternity and nursery phases [35, 36].

Swine rotavirus has a worldwide distribution and has been reported in Africa [37], Vietnam [38], England [39], Italy [40] and Brazil [33, 41].

Since rotavirus can survive in the environment for a extended period and is transmitted via the fecal-oral route, outbreaks are difficult to control [42].

It affects piglets from the first to the sixth week of life, but occurs with a higher prevalence among animals from 2 to 4 weeks. Infection in neonates is associated with failure of passive immunity due to insufficient colostrum intake or the occurrence of a genotype different from that which occurs endemically in the herd [41, 43].

In pigs, the infection is characterized by vomiting, anorexia, slimming, prostration, diarrhea of liquid or pasty consistency and whitish coloration, which lasts for 2–5 days, and dehydration. In more severe cases, because of episodes of diarrhea, the animal may develop electrolyte imbalance, metabolic acidosis and death [43].

Rotavirus infects enterocytes from the apical and intermediate portions of the intestinal villi, causing lysis of enterocytes with decreased absorption capacity and digestive functions [44, 45].

Both asymptomatic animals and matrices, especially in the period of peri-parto, eliminate rotavirus in the environment and can be considered sources of infection [43].

Rotavirus particles are easily visualized by electron microscopy techniques (negative staining (**Figure 4**) and immune electron microscopy), considering that they are present in large quantities in feces and intestinal fragments of infected pigs. These techniques have been used in many studies of the swine rotavirus [46–48].

Inadequate management practices tend to increase the frequency of rotavirus diarrhea. These include weaning in younger animals, breeding pigs at multiple sites, and larger herds have a higher incidence of RV infection due to variation in the immunity level of females [49].

Delivery assistance and breastfeeding management are essential for newborn piglets to receive passive neutralizing antibodies through the ingestion of colostrum, which is the main form of protection of the newly born piglet against rotavirus.

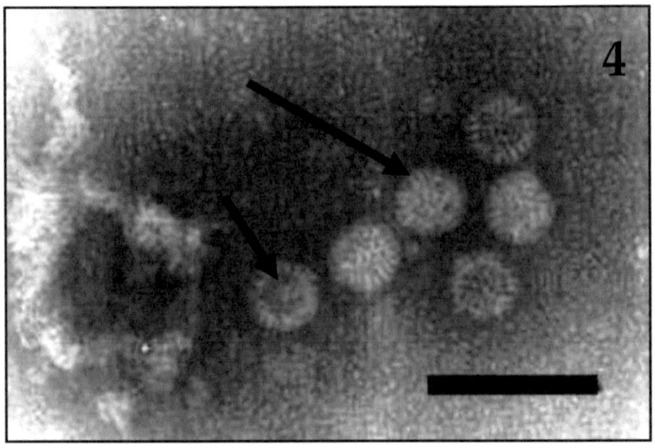

Figure 4. Negatively-stained rotavirus, showing "complete" (big arrow) and "empty" (minor arrow) particles in feces of swine. Bar: 150 nm.

As with all viruses, there is no specific treatment for rotavirus. Treatment consists of controlling the progression of the clinical picture with the use of supportive therapy (electrolyte replacement) and of the secondary bacterial infections with the use of broad-spectrum antimicrobials [43].

1.1.3. Equine rotavirus

Group A equine rotavirus (RVA)-associated diarrhea foals represent a main sanitary problem for the equine industry worldwide [50]. It is the main cause of diarrhea in foals up to 3 months of age, and the acute dehydration can incur severe economic burden due to morbidity in studs [51]. Diarrhea associated with rotavirus can also be a serious problem in areas of intensive breeding during the breeding season [52]. The G3P and P14P are the most prevalent equine rotavirus strain [53].

Clinical signs include diarrhea referred to as white diarrhea or milk diarrhea, lethargy, pyrexia, reluctance to suckle and abdominal tympani. Depression and colic are often observed in serious field cases [51, 54–56]. The malabsorptive watery diarrhea leads to severe dehydration and sometimes death, mainly in neonates with failure of passive antibody transference [50].

Transmission is by feco-oral route via contaminated feces or fomites, and the incubation period is of 1–2 days [57]. The virus invades the intestinal epithelium on the sides and the tips of the villi. The brush border epithelium of the small intestine synthesizes disaccharides to monosaccharides, which are absorbed in the gut. Destruction of the brush border villi results in a decrease in the formation of lactase, resulting in the absence of lactose digestion. This sugar remains in the lumen of the gut, osmotically attracting more fluid [58].

Treatment of foals with rotavirus diarrhea are directed to maintenance of hydration and electrolyte and acid-base balance, aiming to reduce abdominal discomfort or intestinal irritation, to prevent secondary bacterial infection and to avoid spread infection to other foals. The administration of oral or intravenous electrolytic solutions, in addition to intestinal protectors, has been indicated as an auxiliary method in the treatment of rotavirus diarrhea. As prevention measures, isolation of foals with diarrhea, use of protective clothing for the handlers, hand hygiene, use of pedilavium, and appropriate vaccination of animals should be adopted [59, 60].

Direct electron microscopy readily detects rotavirus particles in feces and intestinal fragments of foals with diarrhea [61–64].

1.1.4. *Sheep and goats rotavirus*

Rotaviruses A, B and C have been described in small ruminants [65–67]. Reports on ovine or caprine Rotavirus A are available from various countries worldwide, with detection rates reaching 60% and estimated 10–30% mortality [68–70].

During outbreaks of neonatal diarrhea by rotavirus A, prevalence in fecal samples and lamb, morbidity/mortality may be very high [71, 72]. During an outbreak of diarrhea occurred in a dairy herd of goats in Brazil, rotavirus A was detected in 80-day-old animals with watery diarrhea, anorexia, dehydration and death of one of the animals [73]. Rotavirus A has been associated with diarrhea in goats kids [66, 74]. Regarding the occurrence of rotavirus C, little information is obtained in these species [74].

Administration of colostrums is pivotal to protect lambs from rotavirus-induced diseases [75]. The colostrums and milk of ewes administered with an inactivated rotavirus A vaccine 2–3 weeks prior to mating contained high titers of antibody to the virus [76].

1.2. Coronavirus

1.2.1. *Bovine coronavirus*

Due to genetic diversity and their ability to cross the species barrier, the coronaviruses infect many animals species, including cattle, pigs, equines, rodents, dogs, cats, ferrets and domestic and wild birds [77].

1.2.1.1. *Bovine enteropathogenic coronavirus*

Bovine coronavirus is widespread in the cattle population, resulting in economic losses to the beef and dairy industry in the world [78]. In both beef and dairy herds, BCoV can be associated with calf diarrhea, calf respiratory disease, winter dysentery, respiratory disease in adult cattle, and combined pneumonia and diarrhea in calves and adults [79, 80].

Bovine coronavirus belongs to the *Nidovirales* order, *Coronaviridae* family and *Betacoronavirus* genus [9]. They are simple-stranded positive sense RNA viruses, 32 kbp long, which associates with the nucleoprotein (N) forming a nucleocapsid with helical symmetry. The viral envelope of BCoV is formed by a lipidic double layer with five structural proteins (M, sM, HE, S and I) [81, 82].

Morphologically, they are pleomorphic, with radial projections with a form like-club giving an aspect of solar corona and they measure 75–160 nm of diameter [83].

Transmission of bovine enteropathogenic coronavirus occurs by the fecal-oral or respiratory routes, and most often transmission is horizontal and occurs from carrier dam to offspring postpartum [84].

BCoV causes severe hemorrhagic diarrhea, which is sometimes fatal in young animals, and the spiral colon is the host spot for viral replication in the gastrointestinal epithelium, leading to intestinal villi atrophy and osmotic diarrhea [85].

Once infected, a calf can secrete high levels of virus within 48 hours after experimental infection, and this may persist up to 14 days [86].

The clinical signs are represented by yellow to blood-stained mucus-containing diarrhea, which then progress to a profuse watery diarrhea. Subsequently the animals become dehydrated, depressed, weak and hypothermic, and them suckle reflex is loosened. Most of calves recover, but a few develop pyrexia, recumbency, coma and death [79].

1.2.1.2. Winter dysentery (BCoV-WD) in adult cattle

Winter dysentery (BCoV-WD) is a sporadic acute, contagious hemorrhagic enterocolitis of cattle that occurs in epizootic fashion in a herd [87].

BCoV-WD has been reported through the world including EUA [88], France [89], Spain [90], Canadian [91], Italy [92], Japan [93] and Brazil [94].

The incubation period for BCoV-WD ranges from 2 to 8 days [79].

The disease is characterized by a sudden onset of mucous dark, watery often-bloody diarrhea, which is accompanied by depression and anorexia in adult beef and dairy cattle. Mild to moderate signs of respiratory disease have been reported [92, 95]. The outbreaks occur during the winter season and result in high morbidity and low mortality rates. In an affected cattle herd, milk production may not return to normal for several weeks or even during that lactation period, resulting in significant economic losses for the milk industries. Cattle are more efficiently infected in winter, which increases the environmental contamination and justifies the high morbidity of winter dysentery during the cold months [96, 97].

The intestinal lesions are comparable with those observed in calves with BCoV-induced diarrhea [79]. In calves with BCoV enteric infection, viral particles can be detected by electron microscopy in the feces 1–2 days before the onset of diarrhea and for several days after the diarrhea has resolved. BCV can also be found in nasal secretions of calves with BCoV diarrhea. Recovered calves that are apparently immune to disease can still shed BCV in their nasal secretions or feces [98].

Electron microscopy has been widely used to detect bovine coronavirus particles. Typically, coronavirus particles can be demonstrated in fecal samples by direct electron microscopy (**Figure 5**), immune electron microscopy or immunolabeling with colloidal gold particles (**Figure 6**) [27, 98–102].

In cases of coronavirus infection, the most indicated treatment is the symptomatic with electrolytes, antipyretics, antidiarrheals and probiotics, antimicrobial therapy to prevent secondary

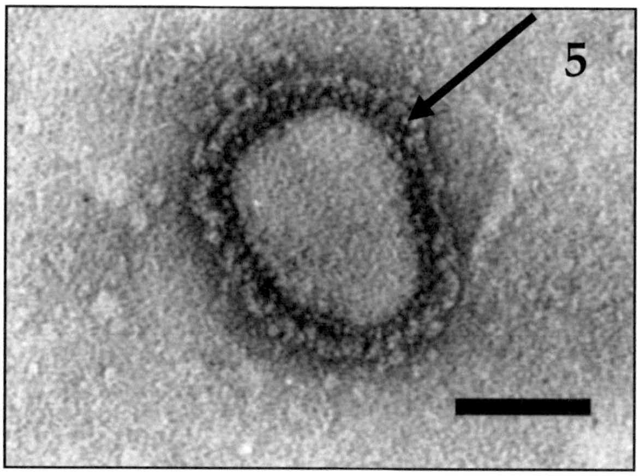

Figure 5. Negatively-stained coronavirus particles containing distinctive club-shaped surface projections, in feces of bovine (arrow). Bar: 100 nm.

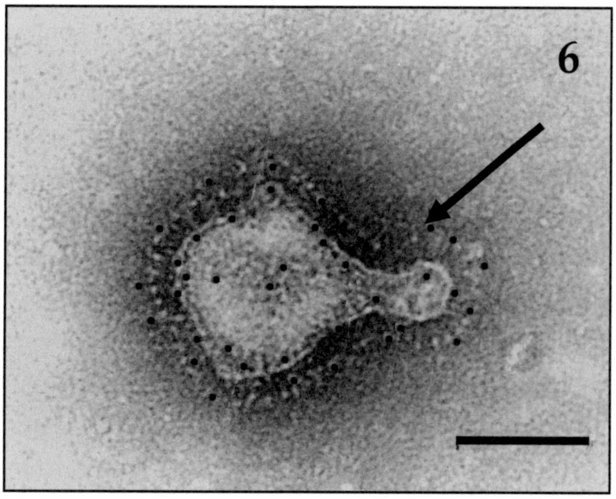

Figure 6. Buffalo coronavirus marked by the particles of colloidal gold (arrow). Bar: 100 nm.

infections, and the occurrence of outbreaks to vaccinate the animals. Colostrum intake has emerged as the natural and most useful method to control BCoV calf diarrhea [103]. The hygiene, management and sanity of the property are important factors for the prevention of neonatal diarrhea, thus avoiding serious damage to the producer [104].

1.2.2. Porcine coronavirus

1.2.2.1. Porcine transmissible gastroenteritis (TGEV)

Porcine transmissible gastroenteritis is a highly severe contagious disease caused by virus of the *Coronaviridae* family and genus *Alphacoronavirus* [77].

As a notifiable disease, the TGEV causes significant economic losses in the pig industry and has been reported in several countries as Europe, American and Asia [105–107]. TGEV was detected for the first time in Brazil through histopathological techniques and the transmission electron microscopy in 19 (25.3%) small intestine samples of pigs from various municipalities in the State of São Paulo and the Minas Gerais, Brazil [108].

The disease affects pigs of all ages, and symptoms were represented by severe watery diarrhea accompanied by vomiting [109, 110], anorexia, prostration, dehydration, dyspnea and death [108].

In the TGEV epizooty, the high mortality rates, up to 100%, affecting piglets of less than 2 weeks of age is a result of severe dehydration [105].

The replication of the virus occurs in the digestory and respiratory tracts, and the target is the epithelial cells of the small intestinal villi that result in the atrophy of the infected epithelium focusing in severe intestinal disorders, which can be fatal in the neonatal period [111, 112].

The transmission route occurs by breast feeding, oral-fecal and fomites [113]. Exportation of fresh and frozen pork contaminated by TGEV allows that these types of food act as a potential source of viral transmission [105, 107, 114].

For the diagnosis of swine coronavirus, the negative-staining technique (**Figure 7**) has been widely used by many authors [115–119]. To confirm the viral strain (TGEV), immunoelectron microscopy (IEM) (**Figure 8**) and immunolabeling techniques with gold particles, performed with a monoclonal antibody specific for TGEV, can be used. Viral ultrastructural aspects can be studied through the resin embedding technique (**Figure 9**) [108].

According to the OIE [107], technique of transmission electron microscopy and *in situ* hybridization was chosen to identify TGEV. Using specific monoclonal antibodies it is possible to differentiate TGEV from the coronavirus that causes epidemic porcine diarrhea and the coronavirus that causes respiratory disease.

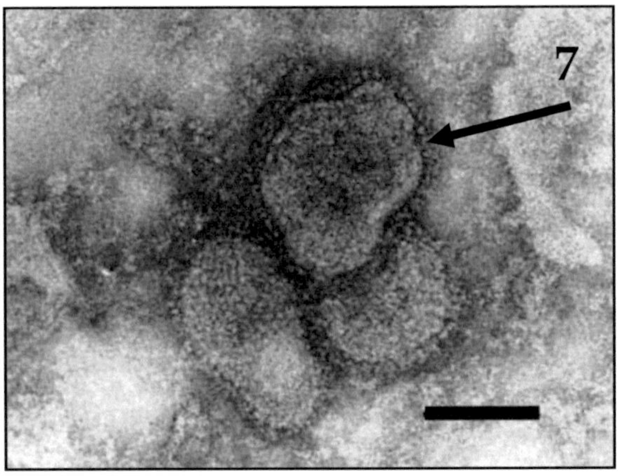

Figure 7. Negatively-stained coronavirus particles, showing characteristic envelope with radial projections forming a corona, in feces of swine (arrow). Bar: 100 nm.

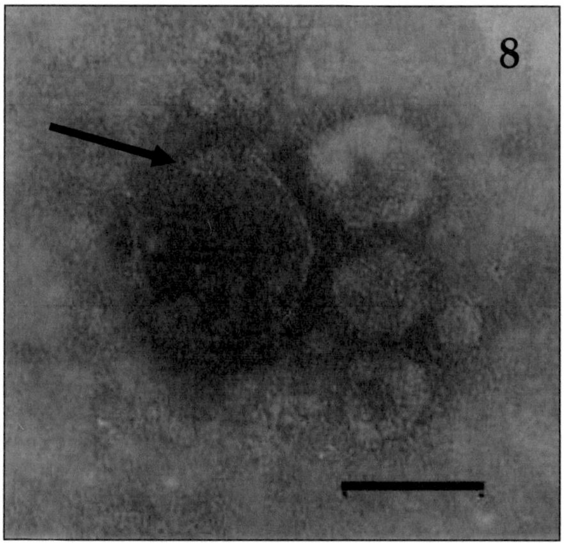

Figure 8. Immunoelectron microscopy of TGEV (arrow) aggregated by antigen–antibody interaction in swine feces. Bar: 190 nm.

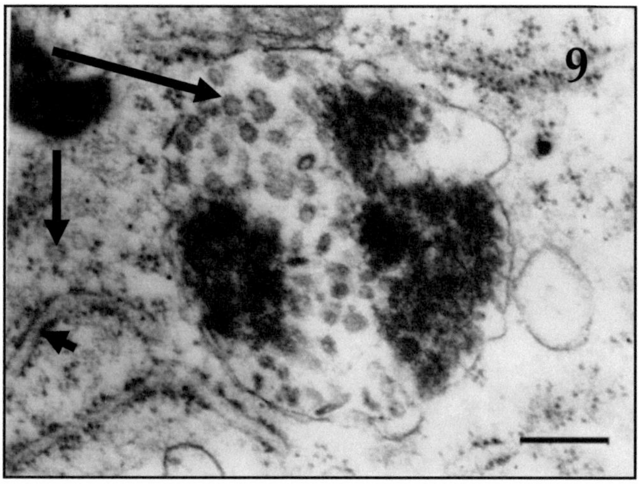

Figure 9. Resin embedding of swine small intestine. Observe coronavirus particles, incomplete, whitin intracytoplasmatic vacuoles (big arrow), complete particle (minor arrow) and dilated cisternae of the rough endoplasmic reticulum (arrow head). Bar: 200 nm.

There is no specific treatment for TGEV. Treatment is symptomatic and seeks to avoid the spread and control of secondary infections, which may aggravate clinical signs. The most important prophylactic measure is to prevent the entry of TGEV in herds [120].

1.2.2.2. Epidemic porcine diarrhea (PEDV)

The epidemic porcine diarrhea virus (PEDV) has been causing incalculable losses to the production of pigs in several countries, modifying the behavior of the swine market worldwide [121].

It was first observed in England, causing a devastating and sudden diarrhea during the winter, leading to losses in pig farms [122]. Subsequently, it was found in Belgium, Hungary, France, Italy, the Czech Republic, China and Asia, where more severe outbreaks were diagnosed. In the USA, it was first diagnosed in May 2013, and during the period from September 2013 to February 2014, losses of pigs in the United States by the swine epidemic diarrhea virus were estimated in 2.7 million or slightly more than 5% of the animals [123–126]. Recently, the presence of the virus has been reported in countries of South America, such as Peru [127] and Colombia [128].

The direct transmission occurs by fecal-oral route. Clinical signs of PEDV may occur within 4–5 days following introduction of infected swine to farms with susceptible animals. Following an outbreak, PEDV may subside but may become endemic if sufficient litters are produced overcome lactogenic immunity. Contaminated personnel equipment or other fomites may introduce the virus into a susceptible herd [121].

The incubation period of PEDV is 3–4 days [129].

Clinical signs of PEDV infection include anorexia, vomiting, diarrhea and dehydration. Morbidity and mortality in piglets less than 5 days is of almost 100% due to severe diarrhea and dehydration, but mortality in piglets older than 10 days is about 10% [130, 131].

PEDV replicates in the cytoplasm of villous epithelial cells throughout the small intestine, destroying target enterocytes because of massive necrosis or apoptosis. These processes lead to villous atrophy and vacuolation as well as a marked reduction in the enzymatic activity, causing malabsorptive watery diarrhea, followed by serious and fatal dehydration in piglets [132–134].

Ultrastructural colon lesions have been observed by transmission electron microscopy. At the cellular levels, PEDV protein E is localized in the endoplasmic reticulum with small amounts being found in the nucleus of infected cells [135].

Although an approved vaccine against the PEDV virus is not yet available, it is important to adopt biosecurity programs to prevent the spread of the disease in the country. These include the disinfection of environments susceptible to contamination, such as breeding, slaughtering and transport facilities, as well as water and food containers. It is also necessary to implement surveillance measures regarding the introduction of new animals in the herd, quarantine procedures and control of access to the farms [121].

1.2.3. Equine coronavirus (ECoV)

Equine coronavirus (ECoV) which causes enteritis in foals is a disease of economic significance in equines for horse breeders [136].

They typically have a restricted host range, infecting only their natural host and closely related animal species but do have the capacity to cross the species barrier to infect new hosts. Equine coronavirus (ECoV) is the only coronavirus known to infect or cause disease in horses [137].

Equine coronavirus (ECoV) belongs to the *Coronaviridae* family and *Betacoronavirus* genus [138].

ECoV was first isolated in North Carolina (USA) from the feces of a diarrheic foal in 1999 [139] and was initially believed to only affect foals. Since 2010, there have been several reports of ECoV-associated respiratory and enteric infections in adult horses in Japan, Europe and the United States, but its global distribution is still poorly defined [10, 140–143]. In Brazil, the first outbreak of enteritis in horses was reported in 1988 by transmission electron microscopy in a horse livestock, in São Paulo, SP, affecting animals ranging from 1 week to 4 months that presented aqueous diarrhea [144]. Later, another outbreak was reported in a farm in Rio Grande do Sul, where 69 foals of 45–90 days were affected by severe enteritis [145].

The main clinical signs presented by the ECoV infection are represented by anorexia, apathy, lethargy, fever and neurologic abnormalities (ataxia, depression and recumbency). Respiratory problems, profuse aqueous diarrhea greenish to yellowish of putrid odor and discrete algia abdominal can also been observed [136, 141, 144–147]. It is transmitted by the fecal-oral route, and signs tend to resolve in 1–4 days, although animals can continue shedding for several weeks [147]. It is suggested that ECoV may spread among horses when they are stabled together or during transport [148, 149].

The virus has been diagnosed more frequently in adult animals over 2 years of age [146, 147, 150]. However, outbreaks have been reported in foals from 5 days to 4 months of age [139, 144, 145, 151] and in both adults and young animals [141].

Morbidity ranges from about 20–57%, and mortality is typically rare [147]; however, a high mortality rate has been described in foals [152].

ECoV has been shown to produce cell death via apoptosis in Madin-Darby Bovine Kidney (MDBK) cell cultures [153].

With the aid of transmission electron microscopy techniques, the disease is more easily diagnosed. Negative-staining technique (rapid preparation) (**Figure 10**) and immunoelectron microscopy (**Figure 11**) has been widely used for direct visualization of viral particles [139, 144, 146, 151, 154–157].

Most adult horses with clinical ECoV infection recover spontaneously in a few days without specific treatment. Horses with persistent elevated rectal temperature, anorexia and depression are routinely treated with anti-inflammatory drugs intravenously. Horses with colic, persistent depression and anorexia and/or diarrhea have been treated more intensively with fluid and electrolyte until clinical signs have resolved. Additionally, antimicrobials and gastrointestinal protectants should be considered in horses with secondary bacterial infection. The use of BCoV vaccine in horses for the prevention of ECoV has not been investigated and cannot be recommended.

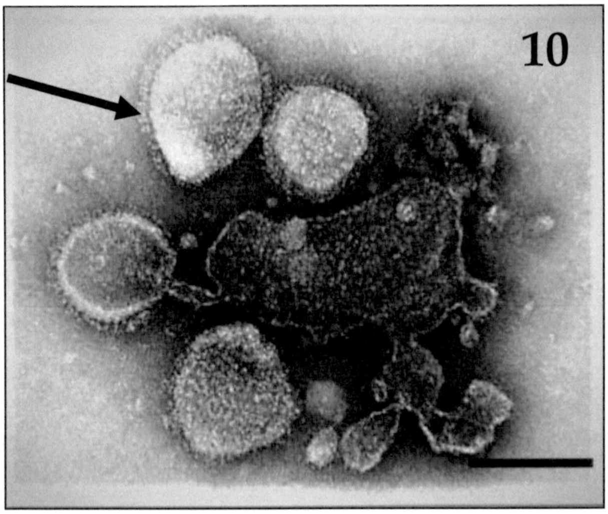

Figure 10. Negatively-stained coronavirus particles (arrow), in small intestine suspension of equine (arrow). Bar: 190 nm.

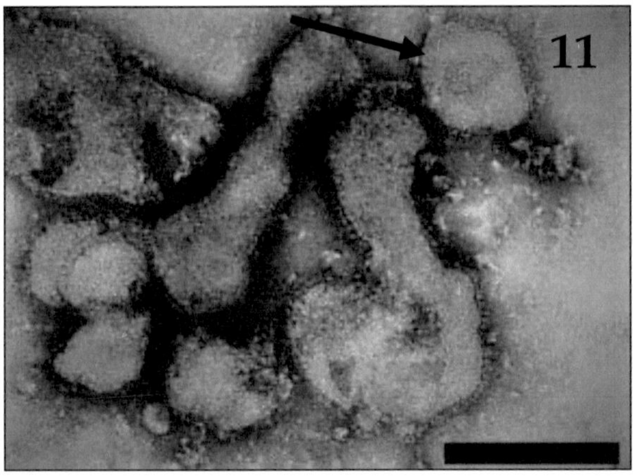

Figure 11. Immunoelectron microscopy of coronavirus particles (arrow), aggregated by antigen-antibody interaction in equine feces. Bar: 190 nm.

The prevention of ECoV infection should focus on the implementation of routine management practices aimed at reducing the likelihood of introducing and disseminating ECoV at any horse-based premise (boarding facility, show ground, and veterinary hospital). Once an ECoV infection is suspected, strict biosecurity measures including footbaths and the use of personal protective equipment should be provided and adequately maintained for sanitary purposes [158].

1.3. Bovine viral diarrhea (BVD)

Brazil currently occupies the position of the world's largest exporter of beef, with the production chain moving around 167.5 million/year, producing 9.5 million tons [159].

Bovine viral diarrhea virus (BVDV) is an important pathogen of ruminants causing severe economic losses to the cattle industry, affecting any productive sector, are it of cut, milk or confinement [160].

It has a worldwide distribution, having already been reported in several countries, such as Italy [161], Australia [162], EUA [163], China [164] and Japan [165].

In Brazil, the presence of BVDV has already been proven in several states, such as Pernambuco [166], Goiás [167], Maranhão [168], Minas Gerais [169] and Rio Grande do Sul [170].

Bovine viral diarrhea virus type 1 (BVDV-1) belongs to the *Flaviviridae* family and *Pestivirus* genus that comprises also the species bovine viral diarrhea virus type 2 (BVD-2), classical swine fever virus (CSFV) and border disease virus (BVD) [8].

The virions are 40–60 nm in diameter, spherical in shape, and contain a lipid envelope [171]. The *Pestivirus* genome composed of a positive-sense single-stranded RNA that is approximately 12.3 kb [172]. BVDV-1a and 1b are the most widely distributed BVDV-1 subtypes in the world and alternate as the most prevalent in different countries [173, 174]. BVDV-1 can be divided into at least 21 subgenotypes (1a–u). BVBD-1i is an uncommon subtype that has been reported in the United Kingdom and Uruguay, and recently, in Brazil [175, 176], and the subtype 1 h strain was isolated in Italy [175]. Bovine viral diarrhea virus is one of the most widespread cattle pathogens worldwide being considered emergent [177].

The clinical signs of BVDV infection are highly variable, ranging from unapparent or mild infection to fatal acute illness. These clinical signs or symptoms include acute or chronic gastrointestinal disorder, respiratory disease in calves, and a hemorrhagic syndrome with thrombocytopenia, skin diseases, immunosuppression and decreasing milk production. BVDV also had been relacioned with infertility, return to estrus, embryonic or fetal mortality, abortion or mummification, fetal malformations or the birth of week calves and infeasible [178–180].

The BVDV induces persistent fetal infection, generating a persistently infected animal with 50% calves lethality rate in the first year of life. The PI animals excrete the virus in large quantity in the secretions, being responsible for the maintenance of the virus in the herd [181].

Mucosal disease affects exclusively PI animals between 6 months and 2 years of age, with a fatal course. The acute form is characterized by a 10- to 14-day incubation period, followed by fever, anorexia, tachycardia, polypnea, erosions in the oral mucosa and nostrils, dehydration, watery diarrhea and rhinitis, nasal and ocular discharge and death within a few days. Animals that survive acute form develop chronic mucosal disease, whose signs are nonspecific [181].

Transmission may occur horizontally through direct contact between animals or indirectly through contaminated secretions, excretions and fomites or vertically leading to congenital infection of the fetus [180].

The introduction of BVDV in the herds occurs by the entry of PI animals on the farms, through the acquisition of cattle during the acute phase of the disease, persistently infected bulls or female breeding PI fetuses and contact between neighboring herds [182].

The laboratory diagnosis is performed through seroneutralization, cell culture isolation, PCR and immunohistochemistry [180].

Bovine virus diarrhea (BVD) particles have been identified by negative-staining electron microscopy (**Figure 12**) in feces, in purified virus preparations, in infected cell cultures and in tissues from infected animals [183–188], being this technique recommended by the OIE for the detection of BVDV [183].

Immunogold labeling technique was utilized for marking BVDV particles (**Figure 13**) and for locating both E (rns) and E2 proteins at the virus membrane [187]. The embedding resin technique was used to study the ultrastructural aspects of BVDV, showing that bovine viral diarrhea virus NS4B protein is an integral membrane protein associated with Golgi markers and rearranged host membranes [189].

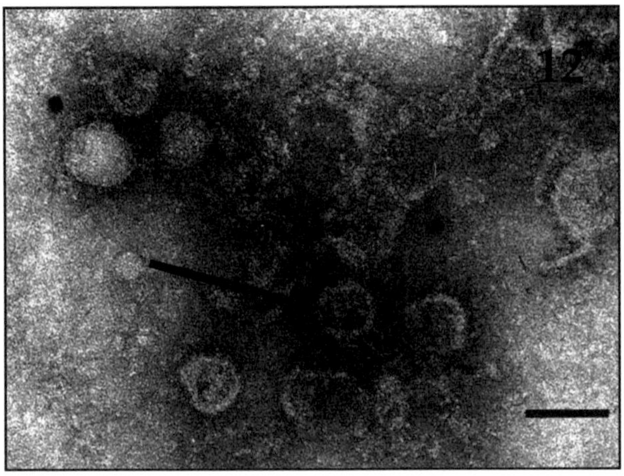

Figure 12. Negatively-stained flavivirus isometric particles in bovine intestine suspension (arrow). Bar: 70 nm.

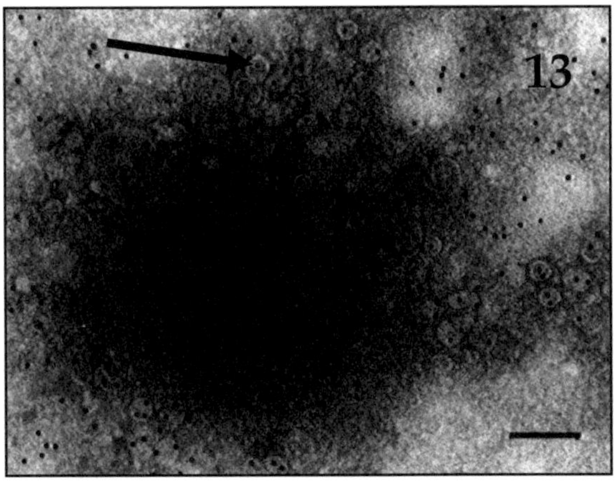

Figure 13. BVDV particles strongly enhanced by the dense colloidal gold particles (arrow). Bar: 140 nm.

The examination of suspected sample by immune electron microscopy procedures is feasible for BVDV virus detection, and it can be used as diagnostic tool, especially for screening of cell culture supernatants infected with suspected clinical specimens. The suitability of this assay for direct screening for identification of persistently infected animals, where the viral load is expected to be high and which are of great concern for control programs, needs to be explored [188].

Considering that BVDV infections cause significant economic losses to farms, biosafety, sanitary and hygiene measures should be implemented on farms to reduce the prevalence of the virus in herds. In addition, quarantine, vaccination and testing procedures should be instituted in the herds for identification and removal of persistently infected animals (IP), minimizing the spread of the virus [166, 178, 179, 190].

1.4. Transmission electron microscopy

Transmission electron microscopy is a perfectly adequate tool to investigate viral agents during outbreaks of gastroenteritis [191]. It is used when it is necessary to apply a fast and reliable diagnostic method to contain the infection and to quickly minimize the animal losses and consequently the economic damages that cause to the rational economic exploitation of the production animals, as much by the decrease of the productivity as in terms of treatment costs. Consideration should also be given to the zoonotic potential of some viruses, such as rotavirus, and the implications for public health [1].

Electron microscopy has led to the discovery of many new viruses, mainly those associated with gastroenteritis, for which it remained the principal diagnostic method [192].

Viruses are grouped into families based on their morphology. Viruses from various families look distinctly, and these morphological variances are the basis for identification of viruses by electron microscopy. The identification to the family level is already sufficient for the recognition of an unknown infectious viral agent and, to allow the immediate adoption of prophylactic measures, control and prevention of the disease [193].

1.4.1. Negative-staining technique

Negative staining has been a useful specimen preparation technique for biological and medical electron microscopists for almost 50 years since its introduction by Brenner and Horne in 1959 [194] as an established method [195].

The technique consists of an electron-dense stain that surrounds the biological specimen and penetrates in the structural crevices to give an image in which the biological specimen appears electron-lucent against the dark electron-dense background. The image is formed by the absorption or deflection of the electrons by the stain, giving opacity to those areas [195, 196].

Due to the simplicity of the preparation of the samples and the rapidity of the results (5–10 min), negative staining has been the most used technique, mainly in the detection and viral identification during outbreaks of gastroenteritis [197]. The large diversity of viruses potentially involved in gastroenteritis contributed to the use this technique in clinical virology [198].

In addition to the rapidity, it has several other advantages, such as to enable the detection of different viral particles in a single sample without the need for specific reagents, to allow the discovery of new viruses, and to require a small amount of sample, besides when detecting the agent to exclude the possibility of obtaining false-positive results [193].

Negative staining can be applied to various types of biological samples. In cases of gastroenteritis, viruses can be easily visualized in feces, small intestine fragments, fecal swab and peritoneal fluid where they are found in large quantity.

Several types of contrasting (heavy metal salts) are used; however, 2% ammonium molybdate and pH 5.0 provide the best contrast to viral agents.

The diagnosis is made by comparing the dimensions and specific morphology of the visualized particles and other taxonomically combined viral families.

1.4.2. Immunoelectron microscopy technique

Immunoelectron microscopy (IEM) technique that consists in the direct visualization of antigen and antibody complexes by negative stain which promotes increased sensitivity in 100-fold, cujo resultado positive, is indicated by the presence of virus-antibody aggregates [192].

The technique was initially developed to quantify plant by Derrick [199] and was subsequently used in several types of clinical samples [200–202].

Immunoelectron microscopy (IEM) is utilized when the number of viral particles in a sample is very low, when virions are pleomorphic and difficult to identify because they do not have a typical viral morphology or when the samples are "dirty" because the aggregated complexes are more easily observed [203]. It allows identification of the virus for specific antigen-antibody reaction and such identification is achieved by its morphology. It is also used to serotype morphologically similar (but antigenically distinct) particles [195, 204, 205].

Several variations of the method such as immune clumping or direct immunoelectron microscopy (DIEM) [206, 207] or immune aggregation electron microscopy (IAEM) [203], solid phase immune electron microscopy (SPIEM) [199] and decoration [208] have been used. Hyperimmune sera, monoclonal antibodies or convalescent sera can be used in performing the technique [193, 203]. The SPIEM has been utilized to detect most of the viruses that cause gastroenteritis such as bovine rotavirus, swine, equine, canine, bovine coronavirus, swine, canine parvovirus and BVDV.

IAEM was used to detect porcine rotavirus (PoRV), porcine torovirus (PoToV) and porcine epidemic diarrhea coronavirus (PEDV) in pigs with enteritis utilizing convalescent sera [203].

1.4.3. Immunolabeling with colloidal gold particles by negative-staining technique

In this technique, the antigen-antibody reaction is enhanced by antigen labeling by colloidal gold particles associated with protein A, using type- and genus-specific antibody. The method also allows detection and identification of antigen structures induced by the virus and its localization in infected cells, serotype viral strains [209], and determines antigenic variants in isolated strains [210].

This technique was used to label TGEV particles in feces and small intestine fragments of infected pigs [108], type A rotavirus and coronavirus in samples from diarrheic calves and winter dysenteric cattle [143], the simultaneous presence of coronavirus and rotavirus in feces of calves with diarrhea [211] and BVDV in feces of cattle with diarrhea [184].

1.4.4. *Immunolabeling in ultrathin section technique*

Immunolabeling in ultrathin sections are powerful tools for detecting and localizing proteins in cell and tissues and to detect virus or viral antigen on the surface of or within ultrathin sections of the cells [195, 212, 213]. The two most widely used techniques are pre-embedding and post-embedding techniques. The pre-embedding method primarily detects determinants exposed at the surface of infected cells such as virus receptors or envelope glycoproteins of budding viruses that are freely accessible to antibodies and reagents. The post-embedding labeling of thin sections allows access to determinants present in the different compartments of the cell and to internal viral structures since they become exposed at the surface of the section [214]. Antibodies coupled to electron-dense markers such as colloidal gold can reveal the localization and distribution of specific antigens in various tissues. The colloidal gold has been the most widely used marker [215].

Immunolabeling in ultrathin sections has been widely applied to elucidate ultrastructural pathological aspects of gastroenteric viruses. Payne et al. [216] studied bovine coronavirus antigen in the host cell plasmalemma in cells traced with colloidal gold particles. Risco et al. [115] investigated the presence of two types of virus-related particles that are found during transmissible gastroenteritis virus (TGEV) morphogenesis, whereas Salanueva et al. [217] reported aspects of the structural maturation of the transmissible gastroenteritis coronavirus (TGEV). This technique has also been applied to check the exploitation of microtubule cytoskeleton and dynein during canine parvoviral traffic toward the nucleus [215].

1.4.5. *Resin embedding technique*

The resin embedding technique followed by ultrafine sections is especially important to reveal fine details of the ultrastructure of all types of cells and tissues [218], and in an infectious process, it allows observing pathogenesis of infection and the identification of the agent [205]. The thin sectioning has the advantage of allowing the observation of virus cell interaction, which reveals the site of virus replication and maturation in the host cells, a pertinent information in the identification of unknown viruses [219].

The ultrastructural set of details not only determines the infection, but also the course of the disease in the creations [220].

Resin embedding technique allowed to study several ultrastructural aspects of the intracellular behavior of the TGEV in intestinal fragments of infected pigs [108] and of the parvovirus in intestinal fragments of newborn dogs with diarrhea [220].This technique also allows studying the efficiency of the vaccines based on in situ produced, noninfectious rotavirus-like particles (RVLPs) [221].

2. Conclusion

The different transmission electron microscopy modalities promote a fast and accurate diagnosis of the different gastroenteric viral agents, allowing prophylactic measures of control and prevention in the creations to be promptly instituted, avoiding animal losses and disastrous economic losses, and collaborating with the National Porcine and Bovine Agribusiness.

Author details

Marcia Helena Braga Catroxo* and Ana Maria Cristina Rebello Pinto da Fonseca Martins

*Address all correspondence to: catroxo@biologico.sp.gov.br

Electron Microscopy Laboratory, Research and Development Center in Animal Health, Biological Institute of São Paulo, São Paulo, SP, Brazil

References

[1] Martella V, Banyai K, Matthijnssens J, Buonavoglia C, Ciarlet M. Zoonotic aspects of rotaviruses. Veterinary Microbiology. 2010;**140**:246-255

[2] Cho YI, Han JI, Wang C, Cooper V, Schwartz K, Engelken T, Yoon KY. Case-control study of microbiological etiology associated with calf diarrhea. Veterinary Microbiology. 2013;**166**:375-385

[3] Zhou X, Wang YH, Souvik G, Tang WF, Pang BB, Liu MQ, Peng JS, Zhou DJ, Kobayashi N. Genomic characterization of G3P[6], G4P[6] and G4P[8] human rotaviruses from Wuhan, China: Evidence for interspecies transmission and reassortment events. Infection, Genetics and Evolution. 2015;**33**:55-71

[4] Svensson CLK, Emanuelson U, Olsson SO. Morbidity in Swedish dairy calves from birth to 90 days of age and individual calf-level risk factors for infectious diseases. Preventive Veterinary Medicine. 2003;**58**(3/4):179-197

[5] Dhama K, Chauhan RS, Maheendran M, Malik SVS. Rotavirus diarrhoea in bovines and other domestic animals. Veterinary Research Communications. 2009;**33**:1-23

[6] Saif LJ, Fernandez FM. Group A rotavirus veterinary vaccines. Journal of Infectious Diseases. 1996;**174**(Suppl. 1):S98-S106

[7] Conner ME, Darlington RW. Rotavirus infection in foals. American Journal of Veterinary Research. 1980;**41**:1699-1703

[8] ICTV2016 International Committee on Taxonomy of Viruses. Available from: https://talk.ictvonline.org/taxonomy/

[9] Matthijnssens J, Otto PH, Ciarlet M, Desselberger U, Van Ranst M, Johne R. VP6-sequence-based cutoff values as a criterion for rotavirus species demarcation. Archives of Virology. 2012;**157**:1177-1182

[10] Chandler-Bostock R, Hancox LR, Payne H, Iturriza-Gomara M, Daly JM, Mellits KH. Diversity of group A rotavirus on a UK pig farm. Veterinary Microbiology. 2015;**180**: 205-211

[11] Uhde FL, Kaufmann T, Sager H, Albini S, Zanoni R, Schelling E, Meylan M. Prevalence of four enteropathogens in the faeces of young diarrhoeic dairy calves in Switzerland. The Veterinary Record 2008;**163**:362-366.

[12] Langoni H, Linhares AC, Avila FA, Da Silva AV, Elias AO. Contribution to the study of diarrhea etiology in neonate dairy calves in São Paulo state, Brazil. Brazilian Journal of Veterinary Research and Animal Science. 2004;**41**:313-319

[13] Bartels CJM, Holzhauer M, Jorritsma R, Swart WAJM, Lam TJGM. Prevalence, prediction and risk factors of enteropathogens in normal and non-normal faeces of young Dutch dairy calves. Preventive Veterinary Medicine. 2010;**93**:162-169

[14] Izzo MM, Kirkland PD, Mohler VL, Perkins NR, Gunn AA, House JK. Prevalence of major enteric pathogens in Australian dairy calves with diarrhea. Australian Veterinary Journal. 2011;**89**:167-173

[15] Cho Y, Yoon K-J. An overview of calf diarrhea – infectious etiology, diagnosis, and intervention. Journal of Veterinary Science 2014;**15**(1):1-17.

[16] AlMawly J, Grinberg A, Prattley D, Moffat J, French N. Prevalence of endemic enteropathogens of calves in New Zealand dairy farms. New Zealand Veterinary Journal. 2015;**63**:147-152

[17] Fukai K, Saito T, Inoue K, Sato M. Molecular characterization of novel P[14],G8 bovine group A rotavirus, Sun9, isolated in Japan. Virus Research. 2004;**105**:101-106

[18] Estes M, Greenberg HB. Rotaviruses. In: Knipe DM, Howley PM, Cohen JI, Griffin DE, Lamb RA, Martin MA, Roizman B, Racaniello VR, editors. Fields Virology. Philadelphia: Lippincott Williams and Wilkins; 2013. p. 2013

[19] Hayashi-Miyamoto M, Murakami T, Minami-Fukuda F, Tsuchiaka S, Kishimoto M, Sano K, Naoi K, Asano K, Ichimaru T, Haga K, Omatsu T, Katayama Y, Oba M, Aoki H, Shirai J, Ishida M, Katayama K, Mizutani T, Nagai M. Diversity in VP3, NSP3, and NSP4 of rotavirus B detected from Japanese cattle. Infection, Genetics and Evolution. 2017;**49**:97-103

[20] Barman P, Ghosh S, Das S, Varghese V, Chaudhuri S, Sarkar S, Krishnan T, Bhattacharya SK, Chakrabarti A, Kobayashi N, Naik TN. Sequencing and sequence analysis of VP7 and NSP5 genes reveal emergence of a new genotype of bovine group B rotaviruses in India. Journal of Clinical Microbiology. 2004;**42**:2816-2818

[21] Chasey D, Davies P. Atypical rotaviruses in pigs and cattle. The Veterinary Record. 1984;**114**:16-17

[22] Chang KO, Parawani AV, Smith D, Saif LJ. Detection of group B rotaviruses in fecal samples from diarrheic calves and adult cows and characterization of their VP7 genes. Journal of Clinical Microbiology. 1997;**35**:2107-2110

[23] McNulty MS, Logan EF. Longitudinal survey of rotavirus infection in calves. The Veterinary Record 1983;**13**:33-35.

[24] Mebus CA. Bovine and ovine rotavirus. In: Dinter Z, Morein B. Virus Infections of Ruminants. New York: Elsevier Science, 1990. pp. 239-244.

[25] Kalkanov I, Dinev I, Aleksandrov M, Dimitrov K, Zarkov I. Morphological and etiological investigations in a rotaviral enteritis outbreak in calves. Kafkas Universitesi Veteriner Fakultesi Dergisi. 2016;**22**(2):309-313

[26] Mohanty SB, Dutta SK. Veterinary Virology. Philadelphia: Lea & Febiger; 1981. 372 p

[27] Athanassious R, Marsolais G, Assaf R, Dea S, Descoteaux J-P, Dulude S, Montpetit C. Detection of bovine coronavirus and type A rotavirus in neonatal calf diarrhea and winter dysentery of cattle in Quebec: Evaluation of three diagnostic methods. The Canadian Veterinary Journal. 1994;**35**:163-169

[28] Schroeder ME, Bounpheng MA, Rodgers S, Baker RJ, Black W, Naikare H, Velayudhan B, Sneed L, Szonyi B, Clavijo A. Development and performance evaluation of calf diarrhea pathogen nucleic acid purification and detection workflow. Journal of Veterinary Diagnostic Investigation. 2012;**24**:945-953

[29] Alkan F, Ozkul A, Oguzoglu TC, Timurkan MO, Caliskan E, Martella V, Burgu I. Distribution of G (VP7) and P(VP4) genotypes of group A rotaviruses from Turkish calves with diarrhea, 1997-2008. Veterinary Microbiology. 2010;**141**:231-237

[30] Alfieri AA, Alfieri AF, Beuttemmőller EA, Brito BG, Médici KC. Aspectos epidemiológicos da rotavirose suína na região Sudoeste do Estado do Paraná, Brasil. Semina Ciencias Agrarias. 1999;**20**:5-11

[31] Paho: Pan American Health Organization. Rotaviral gastroenteritis. In: Zoonoses and communicable diseases common to man and animals: chlamydioses, rickettsioses and viroses. 3rd ed. Washington, USA: Paho; 2001. p. 286-294

[32] Kindler E, Trojnar E, Heckel G, Otto PH, Johne R. Analysis of rotavirus species diversity and evolution including the newly determined full-length genome sequences of rotavirus F and G. Infection, Genetics and Evolution. 2013;**14**:58-67

[33] Molinari BLD, Lorenzetti E, Otonel RAA, Alfieri AF, Alfieri AA. Species H rotavirus detected in piglets with diarrhea, Brazil, 2012. Emerging Infectious Disease. 2014;**20**(6):1019-1022

[34] Saif LJ. *Reoviridae*. In: Mac Lachlan NJ, Dobovi EJ, editors. Fenner Veterinary Virology IV. 4th ed. Oxford, UK: Elsevier; 2011. p. 276-290

[35] Martella V, Ciarlet M, Bányai K, Lorusso E, Arista S, Lavazza A, Pezzotti G, Decaro N, Cavalli A, Lucente MS, Corrente M, Elia G, Camero M, Tempesta M, Buonavoglia C. Identification of group A porcine rotavirus strains bearing a novel VP4 (P) genotype in Italian swine herds. Journal of Clinical Microbiology 2007;**45**:577-580.

[36] Amimo JO, Vlasova AN, Saif LJ. Detection and genetic diversity of porcine group A rotaviruses in historic (2004) and recent (2011 and 2012) swine fecal samples in Ohio: predominance of the G9P[13] genotype in nursing piglets. Journal of Clinical Microbiology. 2013;**51**:1142-1151

[37] Amimo JO, Junga JO, Ogara WO, Vlasova AN, Njahira MN, Maina S, Okoth EA, Bishop RP, Saif LJ, Djikeng A. Detection and genetic characterization of porcine group A rotaviruses in asymptomatic pigs in smallholder farms in East Africa: predominance of P[8] genotype resembling human strains. Veterinary Microbiology 2015;**175**(2-4):195-210.

[38] Anh PH, Carrique-Mas JJ, Cuong NV, ThiHoa NT, Anh NL, Duy DT, Hien VB, PVT M, Rabaa MA, Farrar J, Baker S, Bryant JE. The prevalence and genetic diversity of group A rotaviruses on pig farms in the Mekong Delta region of Vietnam. Veterinary Microbiology. 2014;**170**:258-265

[39] Bostock RC, Hancox LR, Nawaz S, Watts O, Iturriza-Gomara M, Mellits KM. Genetic diversity of porcine group A rotavirus strains in the UK. Veterinary Microbiology. 2014;**173**:27-37

[40] Monini M, Zaccaria G, Ianiro G, Lavazza A, Vaccari G, Ruggeri FM. Full-length genomic analysis of porcine rotavirus strains isolated from pigs with diarrhea in Northern Italy. Infection, Genetics and Evolution. 2014;**25**:4-13

[41] Ruiz VLA, Bersano JG, Carvalho AF, Catroxo MHB, Chiebao DP, Gregori F, Miyashiro S, Nassar AFC, Oliveira TMFS, Ogata RA, Scarcelli EP, Tonietti PO. Case-control study of pathogens involved in piglet diarrhea. BMC Research Notes 2016;**9**(22):1-7.

[42] Qiao X, Li G, Wang X, Li X, Liu M, Li Y. Recombinant porcine rotavirus VP4 and VP4-LTB expressed in Lactobacillus casei induced mucosal and systemic antibody responses in mice. BMC Microbiology. 2009;**9**(249):1-11

[43] Alfieri AA, Alfieri AF, Matos ACD, Lorenzetti E, Lobato ZIP. *Reoviridae*. In: Flores E, editor. Virologia Veterinária. 2nd ed. Santa Maria: UFSM; 2012

[44] Graham DY, Sackman JW, Estes MK. Pathogenesis of rotavirus induced diarrhea—preliminary studies in miniature swine piglet. Digestive Diseases and Sciences. 1984; **29**:1028-1035

[45] Estes MK. Rotaviruses and their replication. In: Fields BN, Knipe DM, editors. Fields Virology. New York: Raven Press; 1990. p. 1329-1352

[46] Terret LA, Saif LJ. Serial propagation of porcine group C rotavirus (para rotavirus) in primary porcine kidney cell culturest. Journal of Clinical Microbiology. 1987;**25**(7):1316-1319

[47] Kim Y, Chang K-O, Straw B, Saif LJ. Characterization of group C rotaviruses associated with diarrhea outbreaks in feeder pigs. Journal of Clinical Microbiology. 1999; **37**(5):1484-1488

[48] Smitalova R, Rodak L, Psikal I, Smid B. Isolation, immunochemical demonstration of field strains of porcine group A rotaviruses and electrophoretic analysis of RNA segments of group A and C rotaviruses. Veterinary Medicine. 2006;**51**(5):288-295

[49] Dewey C, Carman S, Pasma T, Josephson G, McEwen B. Relationship between group A porcine rotavirus and management practices in swine herds in Ontario. The Canadian Veterinary Journal. 2003;**44**:649-653

[50] Parreno V, Mino SL, Garaicoechea L, Barrandeguy M. Equine rotavirus in Argentinean foals: An overview. 10th IEIDC Abstracts. Journal of Equine Veterinary Science. 2016;**39**: S23-S25

[51] Papp H, Lászlá B, Jakab F, Ganesh B, De Grazia S, Matthijnssens J, Ciarlet M, Martella V, Bányai K. Review of group A rotavirus strains reported in swine and cattle. Veterinary Microbiology. 2013;**165**:190-199

[52] Stoneham SJ. Practical aspects of diarrhea in the foal with particular reference to rotavirus and gastroduodenal ulceration. Equine Veterinary Education. 1996;**8**(2):84-90

[53] Ghosh S, Urushibara N, Chawla-Sarkar M, Krishnan T, Kobayashi N. Whole genomic analyses of asymptomatic human G1P[6], G2P[6] and G3P[6] rotavirus strains reveal inter genogroup reassortment events and genome segments of artiodactyl origin. Infection, Genetics and Evolution. 2013;**16**:165-173

[54] Imagawa H, Kato T, Tsunemitsu H. Field study of inactivated equine rotavirus vaccine. Japanese Society of Equine Science. 2005;**16**:35-44

[55] Cohen ND, Chaffin MK. Causes of diarrhea and enteritis in foals. Compendium on Continuing Education for the Practising Veterinarian. 1995;**17**(4):568-574

[56] Fenger CK. Doenças dos potros. In: Reed SM, Bayly WM, editors. Medicina interna eqüina. Rio de Janeiro: Guanabara Koogan; 2000. p. 803-839

[57] Payment P, Morin E. Minimal infective dose of the OSU strain of porcine rotavirus. Archives of Virology. 1990;**112**:277-282

[58] Slovis NM, Elam J, Estrada M, Thao MF, Leutenegger CM. Comprehensive analysis of infectious agents associated with diarrhea in foals in Central Kentucky. In: Proceedings of the 56th Annual Convention of the American Association of Equine Practitioners. Baltimore, USA; 2010. p. 262

[59] Lester G. Neonatologia. In: Savage CJ, editor. Segredos em medicina de equinos. Porto Alegre: Art Med; 2001. p. 247-264

[60] Tillotson K, Traub-Dargatz JL. Gastrointestinal protectantes and cathartics. Veterinary Clinics of North America. Equine Practice. 2003;**1993**:599-615

[61] Conner ME, Gillespie JH, Schiff EI, Frey MS. Detection of rotavirus in horses with and without diarrhea by electron microscopy and rotazymetest. The Cornell Veterinarian. 1983;**73**(3):280-287

[62] Batt RM, Embaye H, Van de Waal S, Burgess D, Edwards GB, Hart CA. Application of organ culture of small intestine to the investigation of enterocyte damage by equine rotavirus. Journal of Pediatric Gastroenterology and Nutrition 1995;**20**(3):326-332.

[63] Ntafis V, Fragkiadaki E, Xylouri E, Omirou A, Lavazza A, Martella V. Rotavirus-associated diarrhoea in foals in Greece. Veterinary Microbiology. 2010;**144**(3-4):461-465

[64] Bailey KE, Gilkerson JR, Brownng GF. Equine rotaviruses-current understanding and continuing challenges. Veterinary Microbiology. 2013;**167**(1-2):135-144

[65] Fitzgerald TA, Munoz M, Wood AR, Snodgrass DR. Serological and genomic characterisation of group A rotaviruses from lambs. Archives of Virology. 1995;**140**:1541-1548

[66] Munoz M, Alvarez M, Lanza I, Carmenes P. An outbreak of diarrhea associated with atypical rotaviruses in goat kids. Research in Veterinary Science 1995;**59**:180-182.

[67] Snodgrass DR, Herring JA, Gray EW. Experimental rotavirus infection in lambs. Journal of Comparative Pathology. 1976;**86**:637-642

[68] Alkan F, Gulyaz V, Timurkan OM, Iyisan S, Ozdemir S, Turan N, Buonavoglia C, Martella V. A large outbreak of enteritis in goat flocks in Marmara, Turkey, by G8P [1] group A rotaviruses. Archives of Virology. 2012;**157**:1183-1187

[69] Gazal S, Taku AK, Kumar B. Predominance of rotavirus genotype G6P [11] in diarrheic lambs. Veterinary Journal. 2012;**193**:299-300

[70] Papp H, Malik Y, Farkas S, Jakab F, Martella V, Banyai K. Rotavirus strains in neglected animal species, including lambs, goats and camelids. Virus Diseases. 2014;**25**:215-222

[71] Theil KW, Lance SE, McCloskey CM. Rotaviruses associated with neonatal lamb diarrhea in two Wyoming shed-lambing operations. Journal of Veterinary Diagnostic Investigation. 1996;**8**:245-248

[72] Luchs A, Timenetsky MCST. Gastroenterite por rotavírus do grupo A: era pós-vacinal, genótipos e transmissão zoonótica. Einstein. 2016;**14**(2):278-287.

[73] Buzinaro MG, Samara SI, Carvalho AAB, Pontes JV, Salles R, Silva DG. Detecção e isolamento de rotavírus caprino do grupo A. Arquivos do Instituto Biológico. 2011; **78**(2):301-304

[74] Munoz M, Alvarez M, Lanza I, Carmenes P. Role of enteric pathogens in the aetiology of neonatal diarrhoea in lambs and goat kids in Spain. Epidemiology and Infection. 1996;**117**:203-211

[75] Snodgrass DR, Wells PW. The immunoprophylaxis of rotavirus infections in lambs. The Veterinary Record. 1978;**102**:146-148

[76] Wells PW, Snodgrass DR, Herring JA, Dawson AM. Antibody titres to lamb rotavirus in colostrum and milk of vaccinates ewes. The Veterinary Record. 1978;**103**:46-48

[77] Woo PCY, Lau SKP, Huang Y, Yuen K–Y. Coronavirus diversity phylogeny and interspecies jumping. Experimental Biology and Medicine. (Maywood). 2009;**234**(10):1117-1127

[78] Kapil S, Lamm CG, McVey DS, et al. Detection of bovine respiratory coronavirus in beef cattle In: Proceedings of the 27th annual meeting of the American Society of Virologists. Cornell University, Ithaca, NY, July 15, 2008. p. 9-10

[79] Boileau MJ, Kapil S. Bovine coronavirus associated syndromes. Veterinary Clinics of North America: Food Animal Practice. 2010;**26**:123-146

[80] Vlasova AN, Saif LJ. Biological aspects of the interspecies transmission of selected coronaviruses. In: Singh SK, editor. Viral infections and global change. First ed. Hoboken, NJ: Wiley Blackwell Press; 2014. pp. 393-418

[81] Holmes KV, Lai MMC. *Coronaviridae*: The viruses and their replication. In: Fields BN, Knipe DM, Howley PM, editors. Virology. 3rd ed. Philadelphia: Lippincott-Raven Publishers; 1996. p. 1075-1093

[82] Masters PS. The molecular biology of coronaviruses. Advances in Virus Research. 2006; **66**:193-292

[83] Cleri DJ, Ricketti AJ, Vernaleo JR. Severe acute respiratory syndrome (SARS). Infectious Disease Clinics of North America. 2010;**24**:175-202

[84] Evermann JF, Benfield DA. Coronaviral infections. In: Williams ES, Barber IK, editors. Infectious Diseases of Wild Mammals. 3rd ed. Ames (IA): Iowa State University Press; 2001. p. 245-253

[85] Gunn AA, Naylor JA, House JK. Diarrhea. In: Smith BP, editor. Large Animal Internal Medicine. 4th ed. St. Louis (MO): Mosby Elsevier; 2009. p. 340-363

[86] Kapil S, Trent AM, Goyal SM. Excretion and persistence of bovine coronavirus in neonatal calves. Archives of Virology. 1990;**115**(1-2):127-132

[87] Tsunemitsu H, El-Kanawati ZR, Smith DR, Reed HH, Saif LJ. Isolation of coronaviruses antigenically indistinguishable from bovine coronavirus from wild ruminants with diarrhea. Journal of Clinical Microbiology. 1995;**33**(12):3264-3269

[88] White ME, Schukken Hein Y, Tanksley B. Space-time clustering of, and risk factors for, farmer-diagnosed winter dysentery in dairy cattle. The Canadian Veterinary Journal. 1989;**30**(12):948-951

[89] Jactel B, Espinasse J, Viso M, Valiergue H. An epidemiological study of winter dysentery in fifteen herds in France. Veterinary Research Communications 1990; **14**(5):367-379.

[90] Abuelo A, Perez-Santos MA. Winter dysentery (coronavirus infection) outbreak in a dairy herd in Galicia (northwestern Spain). The Veterinary Record. 2016;**4**:e000328

[91] Durham PJK, Hassard LE, Norman GR, Yemen RL. Viruses and virus-like particles detected during examination of feces from calves and piglets with diarrhea. The Canadian Veterinary Journal. 1989;**30**:876-881

[92] Decaro N, Mari V, Desario C, Campolo M, Elia G, Martella V, Greco G, Cirone F, Colaianni ML, Cordioli P, Buonavoglia C. Severe outbreak of bovine coronavirus infection in dairy cattle during the warmer season. Veterinary Microbiology. 2008;**126**:30-39

[93] Takahashi E, Akashi H, Inaba Y. Bovine epizootic diarrhea resembling winter dysentery caused by bovine coronavirus. Japan Agricultural Research Quarterly. 1983;**17**(3): 185-190

[94] Takiuchi E, Barry AF, Alfieri AF, Filippsen P, Alfieri AA. An outbreak of winter dysentery caused by bovine coronavirus in a high-production dairy cattle herd from a tropical country. Brazilian Archives of Biology and Technology. 2009;**52**(Special):45-49

[95] Cho KO, Halbur PG, Bruna JD, Sorden SD, Yoon KJ, Janke BH, Chang KO, Saif LJ. Detection and isolation of coronavirus from feces of three herds of feedlot cattle during outbreaks of winter dysentery-like disease. Journal of the American Veterinary Medical Association. 2000;**217**:1191-1194

[96] Saif LI, Redman DR, Brock KV, Kohler EM, Heckert RA. Winter dysentery in adult dairy cattle: Detection of coronavirus in the faeces. The Veterinary Record. 1988;**123**:300-301

[97] Traven M, Naslund K, Linde N, Linde B, Silván A, Fossum C, Hedlund KO, Larsson B. Experimental reproduction of winter dysentery in lactating cows using BCV-comparison with BCV infection in milk-fed calves. Veterinary Microbiology. 2001;**81**(2):127-151

[98] Saif LJ, Brock KV, Redman DR, Kohler EM. Winter dysentery in dairy herds: Electron microscopic and serological evidence for an association with coronavirus infection. The Veterinary Record. 1991;**128**(19):447-449

[99] Heckert RA, Saif LJ, Myers GW. Development of protein-a gold immunoelectron microscopy for detection of bovine coronavirus in calves – comparison with Elisa and direct immunofluorescence of nasal epithelial-cells. Veterinary Microbiology. 1989;**19**: 217-231

[100] Dea S, Garzon S. Identification of coronaviruses by the use of indirect protein-A immunogold electron microscopy. Journal of Veterinary Diagnostic Investigation. 1991; **3**:297-305

[101] Saif LJ, Redman DR, Moorhead PD, Theil KW. Experimentally induced coronavirus infections in calves – Viral replication in the respiratory and intestinal tracts. American Journal of Veterinary Research. 1986;**47**:1426-1432

[102] Soltana MA, Tsai Y-L, Lee P-YA, Tsai C-F, Chang H-FG, Wang H-TT, Wilkes RP. Comparison of electron microscopy, ELISA, real time RT-PCR and insulated isothermal RT-PCR for the detection of rotavirus group A (RVA) in feces of different animal species. Journal of Virological Methods. 2016;**235**:99-104

[103] Cortese VS. Neonatal immunology. The Veterinary Clinics of North America. Food Animal Practice. 2009;**25**(1):221-227

[104] Radostits OM, Blood DC, Gay CC. Clínica Veterinária. Um tratado de doenças dos bovinos, ovinos, suínos, caprinos e eqüinos. 9th ed. Guanabara Koogan: Rio de Janeiro; 2002. p. 1737

[105] Saif LJ, Wesley RD. Transmissible gastroenteritis and porcine respiratory coronavirus. In: Straw BE, editor. Diseases of Swine. 8th ed. 1999. p. 295-325

[106] Sestak K, Saif LJ. Porcine coronavirus. In: Trends in Emerging Viral Infection of Swine. Ames: Iowa State Press; 2002. p. 321-330

[107] OIE. Manual of diagnostic tests & vacines for terrestrial animals. In: Transmissible Gastroenteritis. 6th ed. Paris: França; 2008. p. 1153-1163

[108] Martins AMCRPF, Bersano JG, Ogata R, Amante G, Nastari BDB, Catroxo MHB. Diagnosis to detect porcine transmissible gastroenteritis virus (TGEV) by optical and transmission electron microscopy techniques. International Journal of Morphology. 2013;**31**(2):706-715

[109] Wyllie AH, Morris RG, Smith AL, Dunlop D. Chromatin cleavage in apoptosis: Association with condensed chromatin morphology and dependence on molecular synthesis. The Journal of Pathology. 1984;**142**:67-77

[110] Sur J–H, Doster AR, Osorio FA. Apoptosis induced in vivo during acute infection by porcine reproductive and respiratory syndrome virus. Veterinary Pathology. 1998; **35**:506-514

[111] Haelterman EO. On the pathogenesis of transmissible gastroenteritis of swine. Journal of the American Veterinary Medical Association. 1972;**160**:534-540

[112] Kemeny LJ, Wiltsey VL, Riley JL. Upper respiratory infection of lactating sows with transmissible gastroenteritis virus following contact exposure to infected piglets. The Cornell Veterinarian. 1975;**65**:352-362

[113] Saif LJ, Sestak K. Transmissible gastroenteritis virus and porcine respiratory coronavirus. In: Straw BE et al., editors. Diseases of Swine. 9th ed. Ames, Iowa: Blackwell Publishing; 2006. p. 489-516

[114] Geering WA, Forman AJ, Nunn MJ. Exotic Diseases of Animals: A Field Guide for Australian Veterinarians. Canberra: Australian Government Publishing; 1995. p. 252-258

[115] Risco C, Anton IM, Suné C, Pedregosa AM, Martin-Alonso JM, Parra F, Carrascosa JL, Enjuanes L. Membrane protein molecules of transmissible gastroenteritis coronavirus also expose the carboxy-terminal region on the external surface of the virion. Journal of Virology. 1995;**69**(9):5269-5277

[116] Cappellaro CEMPDM, Bersano JG, Catroxo MHB, Mueller SBK. Presença de coronavirus associado a surto de gastroenterite em suínos no município de Mairinque, SP, no ano de 1988. Arquivos do Instituto Biológico. 1998;**65**(2):111-116

[117] Bersano JG, Castro AMMG, Brandão PE, Villalobos EMC, Cortez A, Soares RM, Ruiz VLA, Leomil H, Catroxo MHB, Monteiro RM, Ogata RA, Richtzenhain LJ. Detecção mista por circovírus suíno (PCV) e coronavírus em suíno: Relato de caso. Arquivos do Instituto Biológico. 2003;**70**(Suppl. 3):75

[118] Barrera-Vale M, Landa HAD, Beiras AMA, Portal AC, Batista ER, Redondo AV, Varela RU, Lepoureau MTF. Transmissible gastroenteritis in Cuba: Experimental reproduction of the disease and molecular characterization of the virus. Spanish Journal of Agricultural Research 2005;**3**(3):267-274.

[119] Nogales A, Márquez-Jurado S, Galán C, Enjuanes L, Almazán F. Transmissible gastroenteritis coronavirus RNA-dependent RNA polymerase and nonstructural proteins 2, 3, and 8 are incorporated into viral particles. Journal of Virology. 2012;**86**(2):1261-1266

[120] Sobestiansky J, Barcellos DESN, Morés N, Oliveira SJ, Carvalho LFOS, Moreno AM, Roehe PM. Clínica e patologia suína. Goiânia: Art 3 Impressos Especiais; 1999. p. 402

[121] Pospischil A, Stuedli A, Kiupel M. Diagnostic notes update on porcine epidemic diarrhoea. Journal of Swine Health and Production. 2002;**10**:81-85

[122] Wood EN. An apparently new syndrome of porcine epidemic diarrhoea. The Veterinary Record. 1977;**100**:243-244

[123] Cui X. Studies on the detection of porcine epidemic diarrhea virus by immunofluorescent techniques. Chinese Journal of Preventive Veterinary Medicine. 1990;**5**:20-24

[124] Fan H, Zhang J, Ye Y, Tong T, Xie K, Liao M. Complete genome sequence of a novel porcine epidemic diarrhea virus in south China. Journal of Virology. 2012;**86**:10248-10249

[125] Son D, Park B. Porcine epidemic diarrhea virus: A comprehensive review of molecular epidemiology, diagnosis, and vaccines. Virus Genes. 2012;**44**:167-175

[126] Wang L, Byrum B, Zhang Y. New variant of porcine epidemic diarrhea virus, United States, 2014. Emerging Infectious Diseases. 2014;**20**:917-919

[127] Quevedo-Valle MV. Porcine epidemic diarrhea outbreak in Peru. In: International Conference on Swine Enteric Coronavirus Diseases. Chicago, IL, USA; Sep 23-25, 2014

[128] Piñeros R, Galvis JDM. Coronavirus en porcinos: importancia y presentación del virus de la diarrhea epidêmica porcina (PEDV) en Colombia. Revista de Medicina Veterinaria. 2015;**29**:73-89

[129] Harris HDL. Porcine Epidemic Diarrhea. The Merck Manual. Merck, Sharpe and Dohme Corp. Kenilworth, NJ, USA: Iowa State University; 2012

[130] Dastjerdi A, Carr J, Ellis R, Steinbach F, Williamson S. Porcine epidemic diarrhea virus among farmed pigs. Ukraine Emerging Infectious Diseases. 2015;**21**:2235-2237

[131] Lee C. Porcine epidemic diarrhea virus: An emerging and re-emerging epizootic swine virus. Virology Journal. 2015;**12**:193

[132] Ducatelle R, Coussement W, Debouck P, Hoorens J. Pathology of experimental CV777coronavirus enteritis in piglets. II. Electron microscopic study. Veterinary Pathology. 1982;**19**:57-66

[133] Saif LJ, Pensaert MD, Sestak K, Yeo SG, Jung K. Coronaviruses. In: Zimmerman JJ, Karriker LA, Ramirez A, Schwartz KJ, Stevenson CW, editors. Diseases of Swine. 10th ed. Hoboken, NJ: Whiley-Blackwell; 2012. pp. 1081-1091.

[134] Kim Y, Lee C. Porcine epidemic diarrhea virus induces caspase-independent apoptosis through activation of mitochondrial apoptosis-inducing factor. Virology. 2014; **460-461**(1):180-193

[135] Xu J, Guo H-C, Wei Y-Q, Dong H, Han S-C, Ao D, Sun D-H, Wang H-M, Cao S-Z, Sun S-Q. Self-assembly of virus-like particles of canine parvovirus capsid protein expressed from *Escherichia coli* and application as virus-like particle vaccine. Applied Microbiology and Biotechnology. 2014;**98**:3529-3538

[136] Dhama K, Pawaiya RVS, Chakraborty S, Tiwari R, Saminathan M, Verma AK. Coronavirus infection in equines: A review. Asian Journal of Animal and Veterinary Advances. 2014;**9**(3):167-176

[137] Balasuriya UBR. *Coronaviridae*. In: McVey DS, Kennedy M, Chengappa MM, editors. Veterinary Microbiology. 3rd ed. Ames, IA: Wiley-Blackwell; 2013. p. 456-473

[138] Zhang J, Guy JS, Snijder EJ, Denniston DA, Timoney P, Balasuriya UB. Genomic characterization of equine coronavirus. Virology. 2007;**369**:92-104

[139] Guy JS, Breslin JJ, Breuhaus B, Vivrette S, Smith LG. Characterization of a coronavirus isolated from a diarrheic foal. Journal of Clinical Microbiology. 2000;**38**:4523-4526

[140] Oue Y, Morita Y, Kondo T, Nemoto M. Epidemic of equine coronavirus at Obihiro Race course, Hokkaido, Japan in 2012. Journal of Veterinary Medical Science. 2013;**75**:261-1265

[141] Miszczak F, Tesson V, Kin N, Dina J, Balasuriya UB, Pronost S, Vabret A. First detection of equine coronavirus (ECoV) in Europe. Veterinary Microbiology. 2014;**171**:206-209

[142] Pusterla N, Holzenkaempfer N, Mapes S, Kass P. Prevalence of equine coronavirus in nasal secretions from horses with fever and upper respiratory tract infection. The Veterinary Record. 2015;**177**:289

[143] Kooijman LJ, Mapes SM, Pusterla N. Development of an equine coronavirus-specific enzyme-linked immunosorbent assay to determine serologic responses in naturally infected horses. Journal of Veterinary Diagnostic Investigation. 2016;**28**:414-418

[144] Cappellaro CEMPDM, Catroxo MHB, Suga O, Mueller SBK, Oliveira JM, Carrascosa AATA, Scatolini CM. Presença de coronavírus em surto de enterite em eqüinos. O Biologico. 1988;**54**(7/12):49-51

[145] Meirelles MG, Araújo LL, Friedrich Junior F, Flores EF, Nogueira CEW. Enterite associada à infecção por coronavírus em potros puro sangue inglês em um haras no Rio Grande do Sul. Arquivos do Instituto Biológico. 2011;**78**(4):605-608

[146] Oue Y, Ishihara R, Edamatsu H, Morita Y, Yoshida M, Yoshima M, Hatama S, Murakami K, Kanno T. Isolation of an equine coronavirus from adult horses with pyrogenic and enteric disease and its antigenic and genomic characterization in comparison with the NC99 strain. Veterinary Microbiology. 2011;**150**:41-48

[147] Pusterla N, Mapes S, Wademan C, White A, Ball R, Sapp K, Burns P, Ormond C, Butterworth K, Bartol J, Magdesian KG. Emerging outbreaks associated with equine coronavirus in adult horses. Veterinary Microbiology. 2013;**162**:228-231

[148] Imagawa H, Fukunaga Y, Kamada M. Detection of neutralizing antibody against calf diarrheal coronavirus in horse serum. Bulletin of Equine Research Institute. 1990; **27**:25-30

[149] Anzai T, Fukunaga Y, Matsumura T, Imagawa H, Oikawa M. Serological examination for viral infection among young racehorses transported by vehicle over a long distance. Journal of Equine Science. 2001;**12**:135-137

[150] Hemida MG, Chu DK, Perera RA, Ko RL, So RT, Ng BC, Chan SM, Chu S, Alnaeem AA, Alhammadi MA, Webby RJ, Poon LL, Balasuriya UB, Peiris M. Coronavirus infections in horses in Saudi Arabia and Oman. Transboundary and Emerging Diseases. 2017:1-11

[151] Daves E, Rush BR, Cox J. Neonatal enterocolitis associated with coronavirus infection in a foal: A case report. Journal of Veterinary Diagnostic Investigation. 2000;**12**:153-156

[152] Ward ACS, Evermann JF, Reed SM. Presence of coronavirus in diarrheic foals. Veterinary Medicine, Small Animal Clinician. 1983;**78**:563-565

[153] Suzuki K, Matsui Y, Miuraa Y, Sentsui H. Equine coronavirus induces apoptosis in cultured cells. Veterinary Microbiology. 2008;**129**:390-395

[154] Traub-Dargtz JL, Gay CC, Evermann JF, Ward AC, Zeglen ME, Gallina AM, Salman MD. Epidemiologic survey of diarrhea in foals. Journal of the American Veterinary Medical Association. 1988;**192**:1553-1556

[155] Dwyer RM, Powell DG, Roberts W, Donahue M, Lyons ET, Osborne M, Woode GA. study of the etiology and control of infectious diarrhea among foals in central Kentucky. Proceedings of the American Association of Equine Practitioners. 1990;**36**:337-355

[156] Mair TS, Taylor FGR, Harbour DA, Pearson GR. Concurrent cryptosporidium and coronavirus infections in an Arabian foal with combined immunodeficiency syndrome. The Veterinary Record. 1990;**126**:127-130

[157] Browning GF, Chalmers RM, Snodgrass DR, Batt RM, Hart CA, Ormarod SE, Leadon D, Stoneham SJ, Rossdale PD. The prevalence of enteric pathogens in diarrhoeic thoroughbred foals in Britain and Ireland. Equine Veterinary Journal. 1991;**23**(6):405-409

[158] Pusterla N, Vin R, Leutenegger C, Mittel LD, Divers TJ. Equine coronavirus: An emerging enteric virus of adult horses. Equine Veterinary Education. 2016;**28**(4):216-223

[159] CNA, 2016. Available from: http://www.cnabrasil.org.br/noticias/brasil-pode-se-tornar-o-maior-produtor-de-carne-bovina-do-mundo.

[160] Bauermann FV, Harmon A, Flores EF, Falkenberg SM, Reecy JM, Ridpath JF. In vitro neutralization of HoBi-like viruses by antibodies in serum of cattle immunized with inactivated or modified live vaccines of bovine viral diarrhea viruses 1 and 2. Veterinary Microbiology. 2013;**166**(1-2):242-245

[161] Bazzucchi M, Bertolotti L, Giammarioli M, Rossi E, Petrini S, Rosati S, De Miaa GM. Complete genome sequence of a bovine viral diarrhea virus subgenotype 1g strain isolated in Italy. Genome Announcements. 2017;**5**(7):1-2

[162] Evans CA, Lanyon SR, Reichel MP. Investigation of AGID and two commercial ELISAs for the detection of bovine viral diarrhea virus-specific antibodies in sheep serum. Journal of Veterinary Diagnostic Investigation. 2017;**29**(2):181-185

[163] Darweesh MF, Rajput MKS, Braun LJ, Ridpath JF, Neill JD, Chase C. Characterization of the cytopathic BVDV strains isolated from 13 mucosal disease cases arising in a cattle herd. Virus Research. 2015;**195**:141-147

[164] Gao S, Du J, Tian Z, Xing S, Luo J, Liu G, Chang H, Yin H. Genome sequence of a subgenotype 1a bovine viral diarrhea virus in China. Genome Announcements. 2016; **4**(6):1-2

[165] Sato A, Tateishi K, Shinohora M, Naoi Y, Shiokawa M, Aoki H, Omori K, Mizutani T, Shirai J, Nagai M. Complete genome sequencing of bovine viral diarrhea Virus 1, subgenotypes 1n and 1o. Genome Announcements. 2016;**4**(1):e01744-15

[166] Rêgo MJP, Batista Filho AFB, Oliveira PRF, Borges JM, França CAB, Ribeiro CP, Pituco EM, Pinheiro Junior JW. Epidemiological analysis of infection by the bovine viral diarrhea virus on family farms in Brazil. Ciências Agrárias. 2016;**37**(6):4119-4130

[167] Brito WMED, Souza WJ, Vieira S, Linhares DCL, Barbosa ACVC, Alfaia BT. Serological study on bovine viral diarrhea in nonvaccinated dairy herds with reproductive disorders from Goiás. Virus Reviews & Research. 2002;**7**(1):144

[168] Chaves NP, Bezerra DC, Sousa VE, Santos HP, Pereira HM. Frequência de anticorpos e fatores de risco para a infecção pelo vírus da diarreia viral bovina em fêmeas bovinas leiteiras não vacinadas na região amazônica maranhense, Brasil. Ciência Rural. 2010;**40**:1448-1451

[169] Figueiredo HCP, Vieira PR, Lage AP, Leite RC. Prevalência de anticorpos contra o vírus da Diarréia Viral Bovina a vírus em Minas Gerais, Brasil. Revista Brasileira de Reprodução Animal. 1997;**121**:11-15

[170] Quincozes CG, Fischer G, Hübner SO, Vargas GD, Vidor T, Brod CS. Prevalência e fatores associados à infecção pelo vírus da diarréia viral bovina na região Sul do Rio Grande do Sul. Semina: Ciências Agrárias. 2007;**28**:269-276

[171] Simmonds P, et al. Family *Flaviviridae*. In: King AMQ et al., editors. Virus Taxonomy: Ninth Report of the International Committee on Taxonomy of Viruses. San Diego, CA: Elsevier Academic; 2011. pp. 1003-1020.

[172] Goens D. The evolution of bovine viral diarrhea: A review. The Canadian Veterinary Journal. 2002;**43**:946-954

[173] Vilcek S, Paton DJ, Durkovic B, Strojny L, Ibata G, Moussa A, Loitsch A, Rossmanith W, Vega S, Scicluna MT, Paifi V. Bovine viral diarrhoea virus genotype 1 can be separated into at least eleven genetic groups. Archives of Virology. 2001;**146**:99-115

[174] Ridpath JF, Fulton RW, Kirkland PD, Neill JD. Prevalence and antigenic differences observed between bovine viral diarrhea virus subgenotypes isolated from cattle in Australia and feedlots in the southwestern United States. Journal of Veterinary Diagnostic Investigation. 2010;**22**:184-191

[175] Bazzucchi M, Bertolotti L, Giammarioli M, Casciari C, Rossi E, Rosati S, De Mia GMM. Complete genome sequence of a bovine viral diarrhea virus subgenotype 1 h strain isolated in Italy. Genome Announcements. 2016;**5**(8):1-2

[176] Mósena AC, Weber MN, Cibulski SP, Silveira S, Silva MS, Mayer FQ, Canal CW. Genomic characterization of a bovine viral diarrhea virus subtype 1i in Brazil. Archives of Virology. 1624;**2017**:1119-1123

[177] Peterhans E, Bachofen C, Stalder H, Schweizer M. Cytopathic bovine viral diarrhea viruses (BVDV): Emerging pestiviruses doomed to extinction. Veterinary Research. 2010;**41**(6):1-14

[178] Brownlie J. The pathogenesis of bovine viral diarrhea virus infections. Revue Scientifique Et Technique OIE. 1990;**9**:43-59

[179] Baker JC. The clinical manifestations of bovine viral diarrhea infection. The Veterinary Clinics of North America. 1995;**11**(3):425-445

[180] USDA – United States Department of Agriculture – Animal and Plant Health Inspection Service. Bovine viral diarrhea (BVD) management practices and detection in bulk tank milk in the United States, 2007. Fort Collins, USA: USDA-APHIS-VS-CEAH, 2008

[181] Radostits OM, Gay CC, Hinchcliff KW. Veterinary Medicine: A Textbook of the Diseases of Cattle, Horses, Sheep, Pigs, and Goats. 10th ed. Edinburgh: Saunders-Elsevier; 2007. 2156 p

[182] Flores EF. Diagnóstico laboratorial das infecções víricas. In: Flores, EF (Org). Virologia Veterinária. Santa Maria: UFSM, 2007. pp. 295-326

[183] Ohmann HB. Electron microscopy of bovine virus diarrhea virus. Revue Scientifique et Technique OIE. 1990;**9**:61-73

[184] Catroxo MHB, AMCRPF M, Petrella S, Pongiluppi T, Lopes D. Identification of flavivirus in large intestine of cattle by transmission electron microscopy using negative staining (rapid preparation) and immunolabelling with colloidal gold particles techniques. In: 21st Congress of the Brazilian Society of Microscopy and Microanalysis (XXI CSBMM). Búzios, RJ, Brazil; August 26-29, 2007

[185] Gao Y, Wang S, Du R, Wang Q, Sun C, Wang N, Zhang P, Zhang L. Isolation and identification of a bovine viral diarrhea virus from sika deer in china. Virology Journal. 2011;**8**(83):1-6

[186] Liu H, Li Y, Gao M, Wen K, Jia Y, Liu X, Zhang W, Ma B, Wang J. Complete genome sequence of a bovine viral diarrhea virus 2 from commercial fetal bovine serum. Journal of Virology. 2012;**86**(18):1023

[187] Wegelt A, Reimann I, Granzow H, Beer M. Characterization and purification of recombinant bovine viral diarrhea virus particles with epitope-tagged envelope proteins. The Journal of General Virology. 2011;**92**(Pt 6):1352-1357

[188] Rajukumar K, Karikalan M, Kumar M, Mishra N, Behera SP, Kulkarni DD. Comparison of immune electron microscopy with direct negative staining for detection of bovine viral diarrhoea virus. Indian Journal of Veterinary Pathology. 2015;**39**(3):235-238

[189] Weiskircher E, Aligo J, Ning G, Konan KV. Bovine viral diarrhea virus NS4B protein is an integral membrane protein associated with Golgi markers and rearranged host membranes. Virology Journal. 2009;**6**:185

[190] Bauermann FV, Falkenberg SM, Vander BL, Decaro N, Brodersen BW, Harmon A, Hessman B, Flores EF, Ridpath JF. Generation of calves persistently infected with hoBi-like pestivirus and comparison of methods for detection of these persistent infections. Journal of Clinical Microbiology. 2014;**52**(11):3845-3852

[191] Schramlova J, Arientova SH, D. The role of electron microscopy in the rapid diagnosis of viral infections – review. Folia Microbiologica. 2010;**55**(1):88-101

[192] Curry A, Appleton H, Dowsett B. Application of transmission electron microscopy to the clinical study of viral and bacterial infections: present and future. Micron. 2006;**37**:91-106

[193] Hazelton PR, Gelderblom HR. Electron microscopy for rapid diagnosis of infectious agents in emergent situations. Emerging Infectious Diseases. 2003;**9**:294-303

[194] Brenner S, Horne RW. A negative staining method for high-resolution electron microscopy of viruses. Biochem Biophys Acta. 1959;**34**:103

[195] Palmer EL, Martin ML. Electron Microscopy in Viral Diagnosis. 2nd ed. Boca Raton, FL: CRC; 2000. 194 p

[196] Harris KM, Perry E, Bourne J, Feinberg M, Ostroff L, Hurlburt J. Uniform serial sectioning for transmission electron microscopy. The Journal of Neuroscience. 2006;**26**:12101-12103

[197] Mast J, Demeestere L. Electron tomography of negatively stained complex viruses: application in their diagnosis. Diagnostic Pathology. 2009;**4**(5):1-7

[198] Roingeard P. Viral detection by electron microscopy: Past, present and future. Biology of the Cell. 2008;**100**(8):491-501

[199] Derrick KS. Quantitative assay for plant viruses using serologically specific electron microscopy. Virology. 1973;**56**:652-653

[200] Gerna G, Sarasini A, Passarini N, Torsellini M, Parea M, Battaglia M. Comparative evaluation of a commercial enzyme-linked immunoassay and solid-phase immune electron microscopy for rotavirus in stool specimens. Journal of Clinical Microbiology. 1987;**25**:1137-1139

[201] Humphrey CD, Cook Jr EH, Bradley DW. Identification of enterically transmitted virus particles by solid phase immune electron microscopy. Journal of Virological Methods 1990; **29**:177-188.

[202] Lewis DC. Three serotypes of Norwalk-like virus demonstrated by solid phase immune electron microscopy. Journal of Medical Virology. 1990;**30**:77-81

[203] Lavazza A, Tittarelli C, Cerioli M. The Use of convalescent sera in immune-electron microscopy to detect non-suspected/new viral agents. Viruses. 2015;**7**:2683-2703

[204] Katz D, Kohn A. Immunosorbent electron microscopy for detection of viruses. Advances in Virus Research. 1984;**29**:169-194

[205] Fields BN, Knipe DM, Howley PM, editors. Fields virology. 3rd ed. Philadelphia: Lippincott-Raven; 1996

[206] Doane FW, Anderson M. Electron Microscopy in Diagnostic Virology – A Practical Guide and Atlas. Cambridge: Cambridge University Press; 1987 178p

[207] Anderson N, Doane FW. Specific identification of enteroviruses by immuno-electron microscopy using a serum-in-agar diffusion method. Canadian Journal of Microbiology. 1973;**19**:585-589

[208] Milne RG, Luisoni E. Rapid high-resolution immune electron microscopy of plant viruses. Virology. 1975;**68**:270-274

[209] Kjeldsberg E. Use of gold IgG complexes and human antisera for electron microscopy identification of hepatitis A virus and polioviruses. Journal of Virological Methods. 1986;**13**:207

[210] Patterson S, Oxford JS. Analysis of antigenic determinants on internal and external proteins of influenza virus and identification of antigenic subpopulations of virion in recent field isolates using monoclonal antibodies and immunogold labeling. Archives of Virology. 1986;**88**:189-202

[211] Catroxo MHB, Gregori F, Brandão PE, Melo NA. Detection of rotavirus and coronavirus in calves during outbreak of diarrhea in Dourados, state of Mato Grosso do Sul, Brazil. Biológico. 2007;**69**(2):114

[212] De Paul AL, Mukdsi JH, Petiti JP, Gutiérrez S, Quintar AA, Maldonado CA, Alicia I, Torres AI. In: Dehghani H, editor. Immunoelectron Microscopy: A Reliable Tool for the

Analysis of Cellular Processes, Applications of Immunocytochemistry. Rijeka, Croatia: In-Tech; 2012. p. 65-96

[213] Rosso F, Papale F, Barbarisi A. Environmental scanning electron microscopy gold immunolabeling in cell biology. Methods in Molecular Biology (Clifton, N.J.). 2013; **931**:517-523

[214] Hyatt AD, Eaton B. Immuno-Gold Electron Microscopy in Virus Diagnosis and Research. Boca Raton, Florida, USA: CRC Press; 2000. 448 p

[215] Cheville NF, Stasko J. Techniques in electron microscopy of animal tissue. Veterinary Pathology. 2013;**10**:1-14

[216] Payne HR, Storz J, Henk WG. Bovine coronavirus antigen in the host cell plasmalemma. Experimental and Molecular Pathology. 1990;**53**(2):152-159

[217] Salanueva IJ, Carrascosa JL, Risco C. Structural maturation of the transmissible gastroenteritis coronavirus. Journal of Virology. 1999;**73**(10):7952-7964

[218] Glauert AM, Lewis PR. An Introduction to Fixation and Embedding Procedures and Their Safe Use in the Laboratory. Biological Specimen Preparation for Transmission Electron Microscopy. London: Portland Press Ltd; 1998. 319 p

[219] Fong CKY. Electron microscopy for the rapid detection and identification of viruses from clinical specimens. The Yale Journal of Biology and Medicine. 1989;**62**:115-130

[220] Catroxo MHB, Martins AMCRPF. Veterinary diagnostic using Transmission Electron Microscopy. In: Khan M, editor. The Transmission Electron Microscope. Chap. 15. Rijeka, Croatia: In-Tech; 2015. p. 326-350

[221] Meier AF, Suter M, Schrane EM, Humbel BM, Tobler K, Ackermann M, Andrea S, Laimbacher AS. Transfer of anti-rotavirus antibodies during pregnancy and in milk following maternal vaccination with a herpes simplex virus type-1 amplicon vector. International Journal of Molecular Sciences. 2017;**18**(431):1-26